MW01280062

PRACTICE PROBLEMS FOR DOSAGE CALCULATIONS

Kathryn A. Melson, MSN, RN

Marie S. Jaffe, MS, RN

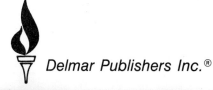

Delmar Publishers Inc.®

NOTICE TO THE READER

Publisher does not warrant or guarantee any of the products described herein or perform any independent analysis in connection with any of the product information contained herein. Publisher does not assume, and expressly disclaims, any obligation to obtain and include information other than that provided to it by the manufacturer.

The reader is expressly warned to consider and adopt all safety precautions that might be indicated by the activities described herein and to avoid all potential hazards. By following the instructions contained herein, the reader willingly assumes all risks in connection with such instructions.

The publisher makes no representations or warranties of any kind, including but not limited to, the warranties of fitness for particular purpose or merchantability, nor are any such representations implied with respect to the material set forth herein, and the publisher takes no responsibility with respect to such material. The publisher shall not be liable for any special, consequential or exemplary damages resulting, in whole or in part, from the readers' use of, or reliance upon, this material.

Delmar staff

Editor: Elizabeth F. Williams
Developmental Editor: Marjorie A. Bruce
Managing Editor: Susan B. Simpfenderfer
Project Editor: Mary P. Robinson
Design Coordinator: Susan C. Mathews

For information, address Delmar Publishers Inc.
2 Computer Drive West, Box 15-015
Albany, New York 12212-9985

Printed in the United States of America.
Published simultaneously in Canada
by Nelson Canada
A division of The Thomson Corporation.

10 9 8 7 6 5 4 3 2 1

Library of Congress Cataloging-in-Publication Data

Melson, Kathryn A.
    Practice problems for dosage calculations / Kathryn A. Melson,
  Marie S. Jaffe.
        p.   cm.
    ISBN 0-8273-4400-7 (textbook)
    1. Pharmaceutical arithmetic—Problems, exercises, etc.
  I. Jaffe, Marie S.   II. Title.
    [DNLM: 1. Drugs—administration & dosage—programmed instruction.
    2. Mathematics—programmed instruction.   QV 18 M528p]
RS57.M45   1990
615'.14'076—dc20
DNLM/DLC
for Library of Congress   90-3790
                                                              CIP

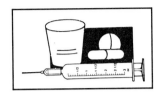 # TABLE OF CONTENTS

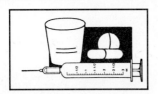

INTRODUCTION

This book was developed in response to multiple requests for practice problems in the computation of drugs and solutions. It may be used as an adjunct to classroom instruction or as a self-paced program. It supplements pharmacology texts and drug calculation handbooks already in print.

Included are problems in the administration of solid and liquid oral medications, intramuscular and subcutaneous medications, intravenous fluids and intravenous medications via continuous, intermittent, bolus, and piggyback methods. Problems range from simple to complex. Medications most commonly encountered in the clinical setting are included, as well as those less frequently found. Actual drug labels have been incorporated into problems to more realistically reflect the clinical setting. Their selection reflects neither an endorsement of a particular product nor of any drug manufacturer.

Each problem presumes the presence of an authorized medical order, whether stated or not. Physicians' orders have been intentionally manipulated to increase the variety and complexity of the questions. Dosages are individualized, and the reader is referred to drug inserts, standard texts, and computer updates for the most recent drug information. Integration of this information into a complete clinical profile is critical to patient safety.

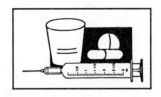

ACKNOWLEDGMENTS

The authors wish to thank

      Ruth Hughes
      Assistant Materials Manager
      Scottsdale Memorial Hospital North
      Scottsdale, Arizona

      Andrew C. Collins, R. Ph.
      Manager, Pharmacy
      Scottsdale Memorial Hospital North
      Scottsdale, Arizona

We wish also to thank those drug companies and manufacturers who so generously supplied the labels used throughout the manuscript.

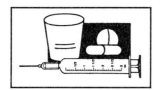

ABBREVIATIONS

IV FLUIDS

D/RL	dextrose in Ringer's lactate
D5 + 0.45 NS	5% dextrose in half normal saline
D5W	5% dextrose in distilled water
D10W	10% dextrose in distilled water
LR	lactated Ringer's
NS	normal saline (0.9% NaCl)
1/3 NS	one-third normal saline (0.3% NaCl)
1/2 NS	one-half normal saline (0.45% NaCl)
RL	Ringer's lactate

MEASUREMENTS/ROUTES/TIMES

ac	before meals
AM	morning
amp	ampule
bid	twice a day
cap	capsules/caplets
cc	cubic centimeter
dr	dram
Gm	gram
gr	grain
gtt	drop
hr	hour
hs	hour of sleep
IM	intramuscular
IU	international unit
IV	intravenous
IVPB	intravenous piggyback
kg	kilogram
KVO	keep vein open
L	liter
lb	pound
m	minim

		ROMAN NUMERALS	ARABIC NUMBERS
mcg	microgram	I	1
mEq	milliequivalent	II	2
mg	milligram	III	3
min	minute	IV	4
ml	milliliter	V	5
oz	ounce	VI	6
pc	after meals	VII	7
PM	afternoon	VIII	8
po	by mouth	IX	9
prn	as needed	X	10
pt	pint	XI	11
q	every	XII	12
qd	every day	XIII	13
qh	every hour	XIV	14
q2h	every 2 hours	XV	15
q3h	every 3 hours		
q4h	every 4 hours		
q6h	every 6 hours		
q8h	every 8 hours		
q12h	every 12 hours		
qid	four times a day		
qod	every other day		
SC	subcutaneous		
sl	sublingual		
$\overline{ss}$	half		
stat	immediately		
tab	tablet		
tbsp	tablespoon		
tid	three times a day		
tsp	teaspoon		
U	unit		
ī	1		
īī	2		
īīī	3		
ʒ	dram		
℥	ounce		

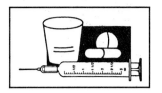 *EQUIVALENTS*

TABLE OF APPROXIMATE EQUIVALENTS		
APOTHECARIES	**METRIC**	**HOUSEHOLD**
1 gr	60-65 mg	
15 gr	1000 mg or 1 Gm	
	1 mg = 1000 mcg	
2.2 lb	1 kg = 1000 Gm	
15-16 m	1 ml = 1 cc	
1 dr	4 ml	
	5 ml	1 tsp
	15 ml	1 tbsp
16 oz	480-500 ml	1 pt
1 oz or 8 dr	30 ml	6 tsp or 2 tbsp
32 oz	1000 ml or 1 L	1 qt

TABLE OF IV FLOW RATES/1 L IN GTT/MINUTE					
TUBING DELIVERS	**4 HOURS**	**6 HOURS**	**8 HOURS**	**10 HOURS**	**12 HOURS**
15 gtt/ml	62	42	31	25	21
10 gtt/ml	42	28	21	17	14
60 gtt/ml	250	167	125	100	83

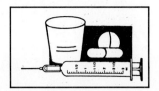

GUIDELINES FOR DRUG CALCULATIONS

1. Essential components of a valid physician order include the following information on an appropriately identified patient record:

   a. date

   b. drug name

   c. dosage

   d. route

   e. time schedule

   f. physician signature

2. Know the drug to be administered. This includes:

   a. classification

   b. drug characteristics

   c. purpose, action

   d. recommended dosage range

   e. methods of administration

   f. side effects

   g. contraindications

   h. laboratory and food and drug interactions

   i. compatibility

   j. potential for allergic reaction

   k. expiration date

   l. nursing implications

3. Conversion from one system to another is approximate. Range selection within a designated equivalency is dependent upon available dosage form and arithmetic divisibility. When calculating equivalencies, a discrepancy of no more than 10 percent may exist between the physician's order and the amount of drug converted.

4. Only scored tablets may be divided.

5. Enteric coated tablets, capsules, or time release medications may not be crushed.

6. Give the least number of tablets or solution.

7. As a general rule, parenteral solutions should be rounded as follows:

    a. to tenths

      i. Round down if the digit in the hundredths place is less than five.

      ii. Round up if the digit in the hundredths place is greater than five.

    b. to hundredths

      i. Do not change if the digit in the hundredths place is five.

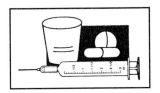 MATHEMATICS REVIEW

Note: The assumption is made that the reader has the ability to add, subtract, multiply and divide whole numbers.

FRACTIONS

A *fraction* indicates a portion of a whole number. There are two types of fractions: *common fractions*, such as $\frac{1}{2}$ (usually referred to simply as fractions) and *decimal fractions*, such as 0.5 (usually referred to simply as decimals).

A fraction is an expression of division with one number placed over another number ($\frac{1}{4}, \frac{2}{3}, \frac{4}{5}$). The bottom number or *denominator* indicates the total number of parts into which the whole is divided. The top number or *numerator* indicates how many of those parts are considered. The fraction may also be read as the "numerator *divided* by the denominator."

Example: $\frac{1 \text{ numerator}}{4 \text{ denominator}}$

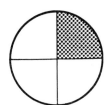

The whole is divided into four equal parts (denominator), and one part (numerator) is considered.

$\frac{1}{4}$ = 1 part of 4 parts or $\frac{1}{4}$ of the whole.
The fraction $\frac{1}{4}$ may also be read as "1 divided by 4."

Note: The *denominator* begins with *d* and is *down* below the line in a fraction.

There are four types of fractions.
1. *Proper fractions* – in which the value of the numerator is *less* than the value of the denominator. The value of the proper fraction is also *less* than 1.

Example: $\frac{5 \text{ numerator}}{8 \text{ denominator}}$ = less than 1

Note: Whenever the numerator is less than the denominator, the value of the fraction must be less than 1.

2.   *Improper fractions* – in which the value of the numerator is *greater* than or *equal* to the value of the denominator. The value of the improper fraction is *greater* than or *equal* to 1.

Examples: $\dfrac{8}{5}$ = more than 1

$\dfrac{5}{5}$ = 1

Note: Whenever the numerator is greater than the denominator, the value of the fraction must be greater than 1. When the numerator and denominator are equal, the value of the improper fraction is always 1; a number divided by itself is 1.

3.   *Mixed fractions* – in which a whole number and a proper fraction are combined. The value of the mixed fraction is always *greater* than 1.

Example: $1\dfrac{5}{8}$ = 1 + $\dfrac{5}{8}$ = more than 1

4.   *Complex fractions* – in which the numerator or the denominator, or both, may be a whole number, proper fraction, or mixed fraction. The value may be *less* than or *greater* than 1.

Examples: $\dfrac{\frac{5}{8}}{\frac{1}{2}}$ = greater than 1

$\dfrac{\frac{5}{8}}{2}$ = less than 1

$\dfrac{1\frac{5}{8}}{\frac{1}{5}}$ = greater than one

Converting Mixed Fractions to Improper Fractions

> **RULE:**
> To change or convert a mixed fraction to an improper fraction with the same denominator *multiply the whole number by the denominator and add the numerator.*

Example: $1\frac{5}{8}$ = (1 × 8) + 5 = 13 eighths or $\frac{13}{8}$.

Converting Improper Fractions to Mixed Fractions

> **RULE:**
> To change or convert an improper fraction to an equivalent mixed fraction or whole number, *divide the numerator by the denominator.* Any remainder is expressed as a proper fraction and reduced to lowest terms.

Example: $\frac{8}{5}$ = 8 ÷ 5 = $1\frac{3}{5}$

Equivalent Fractions

The value of a fraction can be expressed in several ways. This is called *finding an equivalent fraction.* In finding an equivalent fraction both terms of the fraction (numerator and denominator) are either multiplied or divided by the *same number.* The form of the fraction is changed but the value of the fraction remains the same.

When calculating dosages it is usually easier to work with fractions of the smallest numbers possible. This concept of finding equivalent fractions is called *reducing the fraction to the lowest terms* or simplifying the fraction.

Reducing Fractions to Lowest Terms

> **RULE:**
> To reduce a fraction to lowest terms, *divide the largest whole number* that will go evenly into *both* the numerator and the denominator.

Example: Reduce $\frac{6}{12}$ to lowest terms.

6 is the largest number that will divide evenly into both 6 (numerator) and 12 (denominator).

$6 \div 6 = 1, 12 \div 6 = 2$

$\frac{6}{12} = \frac{1}{2}$ in lowest terms

Note: If *both* the numerator and denominator *cannot* be divided evenly by a whole number, then the fraction *is* in lowest terms.

Enlarging Fractions

> **RULE:**
> To find an equivalent fraction in which both terms are larger, *multiply both* the numerator and the denominator by the *same number*.

Example: Enlarge $\frac{3}{5}$ to the equivalent fraction in tenths.

$3 \times 2 = 6; 5 \times 2 = 10$

$\frac{3}{5} = \frac{6}{10}$

Comparing Fractions

In calculating some drug dosages, it is helpful to know when the value of one fraction is greater or less than another. The relative sizes of fractions can be determined by comparing the numerators when the denominators are the same or comparing the denominators if the numerators are the same.

> **RULE:**
> If the numerators are the same, the fraction with the smaller denominator has the greater value.

Example: Compare $\frac{1}{2}$ and $\frac{1}{4}$.

Numerators are both 1.

Denominators: 2 < 4,

$\frac{1}{2}$ is larger

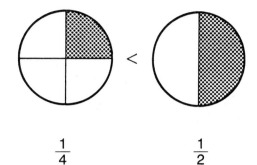

$\frac{1}{4}$ $\frac{1}{2}$

Note: The symbol < denotes "less than," and the symbol > denotes "more than."

RULE:
If the denominators are both the same, the fraction with the smaller numerator has the lesser value.

Example: Compare $\frac{2}{5}$ and $\frac{3}{5}$.

Denominators are both 5.

Numerators: 2 < 3,

$\frac{2}{5}$ is smaller.

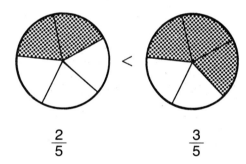

$\frac{2}{5}$ $\frac{3}{5}$

Remember:

- To convert a mixed fraction to an improper fraction, multiply the whole number by the denominator and add the numerator. Example: $1\frac{1}{3} = \frac{4}{3}$.

- To convert an improper fraction to a mixed fraction, divide the numerator by the denominator. Example: $\frac{20}{9} = 2\frac{2}{9}$.

- To reduce a fraction to lowest terms, divide both terms by the largest whole number that will divide evenly. Value remains the same. Example: $\frac{6}{10} = \frac{3}{5}$.

- To enlarge a fraction, multiply both terms by the same number. Value remains the same. Example: $\frac{1}{12} = \frac{2}{24}$.

Review Set 1

1. Circle the *improper* fraction(s).

$$\frac{2}{3}, \quad 1\frac{3}{4}, \quad \frac{6}{6}, \quad \frac{7}{5}, \quad \frac{16}{17}, \quad \frac{\frac{1}{9}}{\frac{2}{3}}$$

2. Circle the *complex* fraction(s).

$$\frac{4}{5}, \quad 3\frac{7}{8}, \quad \frac{2}{2}, \quad \frac{9}{8}, \quad \frac{8}{9}, \quad \frac{\frac{1}{100}}{\frac{1}{150}}$$

3. Circle the *proper* fraction(s).

$$\frac{1}{4}, \quad \frac{1}{14}, \quad \frac{14}{1}, \quad \frac{14}{14}, \quad \frac{1\frac{1}{4}}{14}$$

4. Circle the *mixed* fraction(s) *reduced to the lowest terms*.

$$3\frac{4}{8}, \quad \frac{2}{3}, \quad 1\frac{2}{9}, \quad \frac{1}{3}, \quad 1\frac{1}{4}, \quad 5\frac{7}{8}$$

5. Circle the pair(s) of *equivalent* fraction(s).

$$\frac{3}{4} = \frac{6}{8}, \quad \frac{1}{5} = \frac{2}{10}, \quad \frac{3}{9} = \frac{1}{3}, \quad \frac{3}{4} = \frac{4}{3}, \quad 1\frac{4}{9} = 1\frac{2}{3}$$

Change the following mixed fractions to improper fractions.

6. $6\frac{1}{2} =$ _____   9. $7\frac{5}{6} =$ _____

7. $1\frac{1}{5} =$ _____   10. $102\frac{3}{4} =$ _____

8. $10\frac{2}{3} =$ _____

Change the following improper fractions to whole numbers or mixed fractions; reduce to lowest terms.

11. $\dfrac{24}{12}$ = _____

14. $\dfrac{100}{75}$ = _____

12. $\dfrac{8}{8}$ = _____

15. $\dfrac{44}{16}$ = _____

13. $\dfrac{30}{9}$ = _____

Enlarge the following fractions to the number of parts indicated.

16. $\dfrac{3}{4}$ to eighths _____

19. $\dfrac{2}{5}$ to tenths _____

17. $\dfrac{1}{4}$ to sixteenths _____

20. $\dfrac{2}{3}$ to ninths _____

18. $\dfrac{2}{3}$ to twelfths _____

Circle the correct answer.

21. Which is larger? $\dfrac{1}{150}$, $\dfrac{1}{100}$

22. Which is smaller? $\dfrac{1}{1000}$, $\dfrac{1}{10,000}$

23. Which is larger? $\dfrac{2}{9}$, $\dfrac{5}{9}$

24. Which is smaller? $\dfrac{3}{10}$, $\dfrac{5}{10}$

After completing these problems, see page 251 to check your answers.

Addition and Subtraction of Fractions

To add or subtract fractions all the denominators must be the same.

RULE:
To add or subtract fractions,
1. convert all fractions to equivalent fractions with the least common denominators,
2. add or subtract the numerators, and
3. reduce the result to lowest terms.

Note: The denominators must be the same. You do not perform any calculations on the denominators in addition or subtraction of fractions.

Example 1: $\dfrac{1}{3} + \dfrac{3}{4} + \dfrac{5}{6} = X$

    1. Find the least common denominator $= 12$
       Convert to equivalent fractions in twelfths

$$\frac{1}{3} = \frac{4}{12}$$

$$\frac{3}{4} = \frac{9}{12}$$

$$\frac{1}{6} = \frac{2}{12}$$

    2. Add the numerators: $4 + 9 + 2 = 15 = \dfrac{15}{12}$

    3. Reduce to lowest terms: $\dfrac{15}{12} = 1\dfrac{3}{12} = 1\dfrac{1}{4}$

Example 2: $1\dfrac{1}{10} - \dfrac{3}{5} = X$

    1. Find the least common denominator $= 10$
       Convert to equivalent fractions in tenths

$$1\frac{1}{10} = \frac{11}{10}$$

$$\frac{3}{5} = \frac{6}{10}$$

2. Subtract the numerators: $11 - 6 = 5 = \dfrac{5}{10}$

3. Reduce to lowest terms: $\dfrac{5}{10} = \dfrac{1}{2}$

Multiplication of Fractions

To multiply fractions, multiply numerators and multiply denominators.

When possible, *cancellation of terms* shortens the process of both multiplication and division. Cancellation (like "reducing to lowest terms") is based on the fact that the division of both the numerator and denominator by the same whole number does not change the value of the number.

Example: $\dfrac{\overset{1}{\cancel{250}}}{\underset{2}{\cancel{500}}} = \dfrac{1}{2}$ The numerator and the denominator are both divided by 250.

Also, the numerators and denominators of any of the fractions involved in the multiplication may be cancelled. This is called "cross cancellation."

Example: $\dfrac{1}{\underset{1}{\cancel{8}}} \times \dfrac{\overset{1}{\cancel{8}}}{9} = \dfrac{1}{1} \times \dfrac{1}{9} = \dfrac{1}{9}$

RULE:
To multiply fractions,
1. cancel terms, if possible,
2. multiply numerators, multiply denominators, and
3. reduce the result (product) to lowest terms.

Example 1: $\dfrac{3}{4} \times \dfrac{2}{6} = X$

1. Cancel terms: Divide 2 and 6 by 2

$$\dfrac{3}{4} \times \dfrac{\overset{1}{\cancel{2}}}{\underset{3}{\cancel{6}}} = \dfrac{3}{4} \times \dfrac{1}{3}$$

Divide 3 and 3 by 3 (show "cross cancellation")

$$\frac{\overset{1}{\cancel{3}}}{4} \times \frac{1}{\underset{1}{\cancel{3}}} = \frac{1}{4} \times \frac{1}{1}$$

2. Multiply numerators and denominators:

$$\frac{1}{4} \times \frac{1}{1} = \frac{1}{4}$$

(Product is in lowest terms.)

Example 2: $\frac{15}{30} \times \frac{2}{5} = X$

1. Cancel terms: Divide 15 and 30 by 15

$$\frac{\overset{1}{\cancel{15}}}{\underset{2}{\cancel{30}}} \times \frac{2}{5} = \frac{1}{2} \times \frac{2}{5}$$

Divide 2 and 2 by 2

$$\frac{1}{\underset{1}{\cancel{2}}} \times \frac{\overset{1}{\cancel{2}}}{5} = \frac{1}{1} \times \frac{1}{5}$$

2. Multiply numerators and denominators:

$$\frac{1}{1} \times \frac{1}{5} = \frac{1}{5}$$

(Product is in lowest terms.)

Note: Recall that when multiplying a fraction by a whole number, the same rule applies. The whole number becomes a fraction whose denominator is 1.

Example 3: $\frac{2}{3} \times 4 = \frac{2}{3} \times \frac{4}{1}$

1. No terms to cancel. (You cannot cancel 2 and 4 since both are numerators. To do so would change the value.)

2. Multiply numerators and denominators:

$$\frac{2}{3} \times \frac{4}{1} = \frac{2 \times 4}{3 \times 1} = \frac{8}{3}$$

3. Reduce to lowest terms.

$$\frac{8}{3} = 8 \div 3 = 2\frac{2}{3}$$

Note: To multiply mixed fractions, first convert the mixed fraction(s) to improper fraction(s) and then multiply.

Example 4: $\quad 3\frac{1}{2} \times 4\frac{1}{3} = X$

1. Convert: $\quad 3\frac{1}{2} = \frac{7}{2}$

$$4\frac{1}{3} = \frac{13}{3}$$

$$\frac{7}{2} \times \frac{13}{3} = X \qquad \text{No cancellation needed.}$$

2. Multiply: $\quad \dfrac{7 \times 13}{2 \times 3} = \dfrac{91}{6}$

3. Reduce: $\quad \dfrac{91}{6} = 15\frac{1}{6}$

Division of Fractions

In division of fractions, the divisor is inverted and then the calculation is the same as for multiplication of fractions.

RULE:
To divide fractions,
1. invert the terms of the divisor,
2. cancel terms, if possible,
3. multiply the resulting fractions, and
4. reduce to lowest terms.

Example 1: $\dfrac{3}{4} \div \dfrac{1}{3} = X$

    1. Invert: $\dfrac{3}{4} \div \dfrac{1}{3} = \dfrac{3}{4} \times \dfrac{3}{1}$ No cancellation needed.

    2. Multiply: $\dfrac{3}{4} \times \dfrac{3}{1} = \dfrac{9}{4}$

    3. Reduce: $\dfrac{9}{4} = 2\dfrac{1}{4}$

Example 2: $\dfrac{2}{3} \div 4 = X$

    1. Invert: $\dfrac{2}{3} \div \dfrac{4}{1} = \dfrac{2}{3} \times \dfrac{1}{4}$

    2. Cancel terms: $\dfrac{\cancel{2}^{\,1}}{3} \times \dfrac{1}{\cancel{4}_{\,2}} = \dfrac{1}{3} \times \dfrac{1}{2}$

    3. Multiply: $\dfrac{1 \times 1}{3 \times 2} = \dfrac{1}{6}$

    4. Reduce: Not needed.

Note: To divide mixed fractions, first convert the mixed fraction(s) to improper fraction(s).

Example 3: $1\dfrac{1}{2} \div \dfrac{3}{4} = X$

    1. Convert: $\dfrac{3}{2} \div \dfrac{3}{4}$

    2. Invert: $\dfrac{3}{2} \times \dfrac{4}{3}$

    3. Cancel: $\dfrac{\cancel{3}^{\,1}}{\cancel{2}_{\,1}} \times \dfrac{\cancel{4}^{\,2}}{\cancel{3}_{\,1}} = \dfrac{1}{1} \times \dfrac{2}{1}$

    4. Multiply: $\dfrac{1 \times 2}{1 \times 1} = \dfrac{2}{1}$

    5. Reduce: $\dfrac{2}{1} = 2$

Example 4: To *multiply* complex fractions also involves the division of fractions. Study this carefully.

$$\frac{\frac{1}{150}}{\frac{1}{100}} \times \frac{\frac{1}{4}}{2} = \frac{\frac{1}{150}}{\frac{1}{100}} \times \frac{\frac{1}{4}}{\frac{2}{1}} = \frac{\frac{1}{600}}{\frac{1}{50}} = \frac{1}{600} \div \frac{1}{50} = \frac{1}{600} \times \frac{\frac{1}{50}}{1} = \frac{1}{12}$$

Remember:

- *To add or subtract fractions,* convert to equivalent fractions with like denominators, then add or subtract the numerators.

- *To multiply fractions,* multiply numerators and multiply denominators.

- *To divide fractions,* invert the divisor and multiply.

Review Set 2

Multiply and reduce the answers to lowest terms.

1. $\frac{3}{10} \times \frac{1}{12} =$ _____

2. $\frac{12}{25} \times \frac{3}{5} =$ _____

3. $\frac{5}{8} \times 1\frac{1}{6} =$ _____

4. $\frac{1}{100} \times 3 =$ _____

5. $\frac{\frac{1}{6}}{\frac{1}{4}} \times \frac{3}{\frac{2}{3}} =$ _____

Add and reduce the answers to lowest terms.

6. $7\frac{4}{5} + \frac{2}{3} =$ _____

7. $\frac{3}{4} + \frac{2}{3} =$ _____

8. $4\frac{2}{3} + 5\frac{1}{24} + 7\frac{1}{2} =$ _____

9. $\frac{3}{4} + \frac{1}{8} + \frac{1}{6} =$ _____

10. $12\frac{1}{2} + 20\frac{1}{3} =$ _____

Subtract and reduce the answers to lowest terms.

11. $\dfrac{3}{4} - \dfrac{1}{4} =$ _____

12. $8\dfrac{1}{12} - 3\dfrac{1}{4} =$ _____

13. $\dfrac{1}{8} - \dfrac{1}{12} =$ _____

14. $100\dfrac{1}{33} - 33\dfrac{1}{3} =$ _____

15. $355\dfrac{1}{5} - 55\dfrac{2}{5} =$ _____

Divide and reduce the answers to lowest terms.

16. $\dfrac{1}{60} \div \dfrac{1}{2} =$ _____

17. $2\dfrac{1}{2} \div \dfrac{3}{4} =$ _____

18. $\dfrac{\frac{1}{20}}{\frac{1}{3}} =$ _____

19. $\dfrac{1}{150} \div \dfrac{1}{50} =$ _____

20. $\dfrac{\frac{3}{4}}{\frac{7}{8}} \div \dfrac{1\frac{1}{2}}{2\frac{1}{3}} =$ _____

After completing these problems, see page 251 to check your answers.

DECIMALS

Decimals or *decimal fractions* are fractions with a denominator of 10, 100, 1000, or any multiple or power of 10. The position of the number in relation to the decimal point indicates its value.

Example: Look carefully at the decimal fraction 0.125.

$$0 \;.\; 1 \quad 2 \quad 5$$

Tenths | Hundredths | Thousandths

0.125 = 125/1000 or one hundred twenty-five thousandths
0.125 is less than 0.25 (twenty-five hundredths) but greater than 0.0125 (one hundred twenty-five ten thousandths)

Zeros added after the last digit of a decimal fraction *do not* change its value: 0.25 = 0.250. Zeros added between the decimal point and the first digit of a decimal fraction *do* change its value: 0.125 ≠ ("is *not* equal to") 0.0125.

To eliminate possible confusion by overlooking a decimal as a whole number, *always* place a zero to the left of the decimal point to emphasize it: *0.125, 0.01, 0.005.*

Read decimals by naming the value of the place: 0.1 = $\frac{1}{10}$ is read "one-tenth." In the case of mixed decimals, read the *decimal point* as "and": 1.01 = $1\frac{1}{100}$ is read "one *and* one-hundredth.

For dosage calculations you may need to convert decimals to fractions and vice versa.

RULE:
To convert a fraction to a decimal, divide the denominator into the numerator.

Example: $\frac{1}{4}$ = 4)$\overline{1.00}$ = 0.25

$$\begin{array}{r} .25 \\ 4)\overline{1.00} \\ \underline{8} \\ 20 \\ \underline{20} \end{array}$$

RULE:
To convert a decimal to a fraction,
1. express the decimal number as a whole number in the numerator of the fraction,
2. express the denominator of the fraction as the number 1 followed by as many zeros as there are places to the right of the decimal point, and
3. reduce the resultant fraction to lowest terms.

Example: 0.125 = X

1. Numerator: 125

2. Denominator: 1 + 3 zeros = 1000

3. Reduce: $\frac{125}{1000} = \frac{1}{8}$

Review Set 3

Complete the following table of equivalent fractions and decimals. Reduce fractions to lowest terms.

	Fraction	Decimal	To be read as:
1.	$\dfrac{1}{5}$	_____	_____
2.	_____	_____	eighty-five hundredths
3.	_____	1.05	_____
4.	_____	0.006	_____
5.	$10\dfrac{3}{200}$	_____	_____
6.	_____	1.9	_____
7.	_____	_____	five and one-tenth
8.	$\dfrac{4}{5}$	_____	_____
9.	_____	250.5	_____
10.	$33\dfrac{3}{100}$	_____	_____
11.	_____	0.95	_____
12.	$2\dfrac{3}{4}$	_____	_____
13.	_____	_____	seven and five-thousandths
14.	$\dfrac{21}{250}$	_____	_____
15.	_____	12.125	_____

	Fraction	Decimal	To be read as:

16. _____   20.09   _____

17. _____   _____   twenty-two and twenty-two thousandths

18. _____   0.15   _____

19. $1000\frac{1}{200}$ _____   _____

20. _____   _____   four thousand eighty-five and seventy-five thousandths

After completing these problems, see pages 252 and 253 to check your answers.

Addition and Subtraction of Decimals

The addition and subtraction of decimals is very similar to addition and subtraction of whole numbers. There are only two simple rules that are different.

RULE:
To add and subtract decimal numbers, line up the decimal points.

Example 1: $1.25 + 1.75 =$ $\begin{array}{r} 1.25 \\ +\ 1.75 \\ \hline 3.00 \end{array} = 3$

Example 2: $1.25 - 0.13 =$ $\begin{array}{r} 1.25 \\ -\ 0.13 \\ \hline 1.12 \end{array}$

RULE:
To add and subtract decimal numbers, add zeros to avoid confusion, making all decimal numbers of equal length.

Example 1:   3.75 − 2.1 = 3.75
$$\begin{array}{r} 3.75 \\ -\ 2.10 \\ \hline 1.65 \end{array}$$

Example 2:   Add 0.9, 0.65, 0.27, 4.712
$$\begin{array}{r} 0.900 \\ 0.650 \\ 0.270 \\ +\ 4.712 \\ \hline 6.532 \end{array}$$

Review Set 4
Find the result of the following problems.

1.   0.16 + 5.375 + 1.05 + 16 =   _____

2.   7.517 + 3.2 + 0.16 + 33.3 =   _____

3.   13.009 − 0.7 =   _____

4.   5.125 + 6.025 + 0.15 =   _____

5.   175.1 + 0.099 =   _____

6.   25.2 − 0.193 =   _____

7.   0.58 − 0.062 =   _____

8. $10.10 − $0.62 =   _____

9. $19 − $0.09 =   _____

10. $5.05 + $0.17 + $17.49 =   _____

11.   4 + 1.98 + 0.42 + 0.003 =   _____

12.   0.3 − 0.03 =   _____

13.   16.3 − 12.15 =   _____

14.   2.5 − 0.99 =   _____

15.   5 + 2.5 + 0.05 + 0.15 + 2.55 =   _____

16.   0.03 + 0.16 + 2.327 =   _____

17.   700 − 325.65 =   _____

18. 645.32 − 40.9 =   _____

19. 18 + 2.35 + 7.006 + 0.093 =   _____

20. 13.529 + 10.09 =   _____

After completing these problems, see page 253 to check your answers.

Multiplying Decimals

The procedure in multiplication of decimals is the same as for whole numbers. The only difference is in the expression of the product or answer. Follow this simple rule:

> **RULE:**
> To multiply decimals,
> 1. multiply the decimals without concern for decimal placement,
> 2. count off the number of decimal places in the decimals multiplied, and
> 3. place the decimal point in the product to the left of the total number of places counted.

Example 1:   1.5 × 0.5 =   1.5   (1 decimal place)
                                  × 0.5   (1 decimal place)
                                  0.75   (The decimal point is located 2 places to the left, because *2* decimal places are counted.)

Example 2:   1.72 × 0.9 =   1.72   (2 decimal places)
                                  × 0.9   (1 decimal place)
                                  1.548   (The decimal point is located 3 places to the left, because *3* decimal places are counted.)

Example 3:   5.06 × 1.3 =   5.06   (2 decimal places)
                                  ×   1.3   (1 decimal place)
                                  1 518
                                + 5 06
                                  6.578   (The decimal point is located 3 places to the left, because *3* decimal places are counted.)

RULE:
When multiplying a decimal by a power of ten, move the decimal point as many places to the right as there are zeros in the multiplier.

Example 1:   Multiply 1.25 by 10

The multiplier 10 has 1 zero; move the decimal point 1 place to the right.

1.25 × 10 = 1.2.5 = 12.5

Example 2:   Multiply 2.3 × 100

The multiplier 100 has 2 zeros; move the decimal point 2 places to the right. (Note: add zeros as necessary to complete the operation.)

2.3 × 100 = 2.30. = 230

Example 3:   Multiply 0.001 × 1000

The multiplier 1000 has 3 zeros; move the decimal point 3 places to the right.

0.001 × 1000 = 0.001. = 1

Dividing Decimals

When dividing decimals, set up the problem the same as for the division of whole numbers. Follow the same procedure for dividing whole numbers, after you apply the following rule.

RULE:
To divide decimals,
1. move the decimal in the divisor (number divided by) and the dividend (number divided), the number of places needed to make the *divisor* a *whole number*;
2. place the decimal point in the quotient (answer) above the new decimal place in the dividend.

Note: Moving the decimal point to the right is the same as multiplying by 10, 100, 1000, etc. Recall the rule: multiplying or dividing both sides of a fraction by the same number does not change the value.

Example 1: $100.75 \div 2.5 =$

$$\begin{array}{r} 4\,0.3 \\ 2.5.\overline{)100.7\!5} \\ \underline{100} \\ 75 \\ \underline{75} \end{array} = 40.3$$

(dividend)   (divisor)

Example 2: $56.5 \div 0.02 =$

$$\begin{array}{r} 28\;25. \\ 0.02.\overline{)56.50} \\ \underline{4} \\ 16 \\ \underline{16} \\ 5 \\ \underline{4} \\ 10 \\ \underline{10} \end{array} = 2825$$

Note: Recall that adding a zero after a decimal does not change its value. (56.5 = 56.50)

RULE:
When dividing a decimal by a power of ten, move the decimal point to the left as many places as there are zeros in the divisor.

Example 1: Divide 0.65 by 10

The divisor 10 has 1 zero; move the decimal point 1 place to the left.

$0.65 \div 10 = .0.65 = 0.065$

(Note: place the zero to the left of the decimal point to avoid confusion and to emphasize that this is a decimal.)

Example 2: Divide 7.3 by 100

The divisor 100 has 2 zeros; move the decimal point 2 places to the left.

$7.3 \div 100 = .07.3 = 0.073$

(Note: add zeros as necessary to complete the operation.)

Example 3: Divide 0.5 by 1000

The divisor 1000 has 3 zeros; move the decimal point 3 places to the left.

$0.5 \div 1000 = .000.5 = 0.0005$

Rounding Decimal Fractions

RULE:
To round a decimal to hundredths,
1. do not change the number in hundredths place, if the number in thousandths place is 4 or less;
2. increase the number in hundredths place by 1, if the number in thousandths place is 5 or more.

Examples: 0.123 = 0.12   Rounded to hundredths (two places)
          1.744 = 1.74
          5.325 = 5.33
          0.666 = 0.67

RULE:
To round a decimal to tenths,
1. do not change the number in tenths place, if the number in hundredths place is 4 or less;
2. increase the number in tenths place by 1, if the number in hundredths place is 5 or more.

Examples: 0.13 = 0.1   Rounded to tenths (one place)
          5.64 = 5.6
          0.75 = 0.8
          1.66 = 1.7

Remember:

- To multiply decimals, place the decimal point in the product to the *left* as many decimal places as there are in the two decimals multiplied. Example: 0.25 × 0.2 = 0.050 = 0.05

- To divide decimals, move the decimal point in the divisor and dividend the number of decimal places that will make the divisor a whole number. Example:

$$1.2\overline{)24.0}^{\textstyle 2\,0.}$$

- To multiply or divide decimals by powers of 10, move the decimal to the *right* (to *multiply*) or to the *left* (to *divide*) the number of decimal places as there are zeros in the multiple of 10. Examples: 5.60 × 10 = 5.0̲6 = 50.6; 2.1 ÷ 100 = .0̲2.1 = 0.021

- When rounding decimals, add 1 to the place value considered if the next decimal place is 5 or greater. Examples: (rounded to hundredths place) 3.054 = 3.05; 0.566 = 0.57; (rounded to tenths place) 3.05 = 3.1; 0.54 = 0.5

Review Set 5

Multiply and round your answers to two decimal places.

1. 1.16 × 5.03 = _____
2. 0.314 × 7 = _____
3. 1.71 × 25 = _____
4. 3.002 × 0.05 = _____
5. 16.1 × 25.04 = _____

6. 75.1 × 1000.01 = _____
7. $16.03 × $2.05 = _____
8. $55.50 × $0.05 = _____
9. 23.2 × 15.025 = _____
10. 1.14 × 0.014 = _____

Divide and round your answers to two decimal places.

11. 16 ÷ 0.04 = _____
12. 25.3 ÷ 6.76 = _____
13. 0.02 ÷ 0.004 = _____
14. 45.5 ÷ 15.25 = _____
15. 515 ÷ 0.125 = _____

16. $73 ÷ $13.40 = _____
17. $16.36 ÷ $0.06 = _____
18. 0.375 ÷ 0.25 = _____
19. 100.04 ÷ 0.002 = _____
20. $45 ÷ $0.15 = _____

Multiply or divide by the power of 10 indicated. Draw an arrow to demonstrate movement of the decimal point.

21. 562.5 × 100 = _____
22. 16 × 10 = _____
23. 25 ÷ 1000 = _____
24. 32.005 ÷ 1000 = _____
25. 0.125 ÷ 100 = _____

26. 23.25 × 10 = _____
27. 717.717 ÷ 10 = _____
28. 83.16 × 10 = _____
29. 0.33 × 100 = _____
30. 14.106 × 1000 = _____

After completing these problems, see pages 253 and 254 to check your answers.

RATIO AND PERCENT

Other expressions equivalent to fractions ($\frac{1}{2}$) and decimals (0.5) are ratios (1:2) and percents (50%).

A *ratio* is used to indicate the relationship of one quantity to another. When written, the two quantities are separated by a colon (:).

In drug solutions, the ratio is used occasionally to indicate the amount of drug to the amount of solution.

Example: Adrenalin 1:1000 solution = 1 part Adrenalin to 1000 parts solution.

Actually a ratio is the same as a fraction; 1:1000 is the same as $\frac{1}{1000}$.

Percent means per hundred parts or hundredth part. Percent is a fraction or a ratio with the denominator always being 100. The symbol for percent is %.

Example: 25% = $\frac{25}{100}$ = 25:100 = 25 parts per 100 parts

Since the denominator of a percent is always 100, it is easy to find the equivalent decimal. Recall that to divide by 100, move the decimal point to the left the number of places equal to the number of zeros in the denominator.

Example: 25% = $\frac{25}{100}$ = 25 ÷ 100 = .25. = 0.25

Remember:

- To change a percent to a decimal fraction, move the decimal point two places to the left. Example: 4% = .04. = 0.04

Review Set 6

Find the equivalent decimal, fraction, percent, and ratio forms. Reduce fractions and ratios to lowest terms; round decimals to two places.

	Decimal	Fraction	Percent	Ratio
1.	_____	$\frac{2}{5}$	_____	_____
2.	0.05	_____	_____	_____

	Decimal	Fraction	Percent	Ratio
3.	_____	_____	17%	_____
4.	_____	_____	_____	1:4
5.	_____	_____	6%	_____
6.	_____	$\frac{1}{6}$	_____	_____
7.	_____	_____	50%	_____
8.	_____	_____	_____	1:100
9.	0.09	_____	_____	_____
10.	_____	$\frac{3}{8}$	_____	_____
11.	_____	_____	_____	2:3
12.	_____	$\frac{1}{3}$	_____	_____
13.	0.52	_____	_____	_____
14.	_____	_____	_____	9:20
15.	_____	$\frac{6}{7}$	_____	_____
16.	_____	_____	_____	3:10
17.	_____	$\frac{1}{50}$	_____	_____
18.	0.6	_____	_____	_____
19.	0.04	_____	_____	_____
20.	_____	_____	10%	_____

After completing these problems, see page 254 to check your answers.

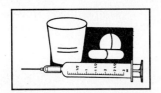

Chapter 1   ORAL MEDICATIONS

1. Metoclopramide hydrochloride 5 mg po is prescribed ac and hs. Ten mg scored tab are available. How many tab should be administered per dose?

2. The physician orders 0.5 Gm of ciprofloxacin hydrochloride po q12h. If the drug is supplied in 500 mg tab, how many tab should be administered per dose?

3. Glipizide 2.5 mg po ac is ordered. Glipizide is available in scored tab of 5 mg each. How many tab should be administered?

4. Quinidine sulfate is supplied in 200 mg tab. How many tab should be administered per dose if gr ꠚꠚꠚ is prescribed?

5. How many scored 2.5 mg tab of mecamylamine hydrochloride should be administered if gr 1/12 is prescribed?

6. Scored 1.34 mg tab of clemastine fumarate are available. How many tab should be administered per dose if the physician orders 2.68 mg po bid?

7. "RX: Chloral hydrate 500 mg po hs." How many ml should be administered if the medication is available in a syrup, dosage 1 Gm/10 ml?

8. Using the information in Figure 1-1, how many tab should be administered if 150 mg are ordered po qd?

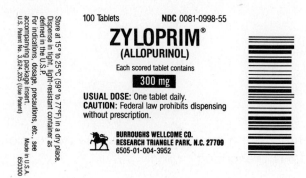

FIGURE 1-1 Zyloprim 300 mg (Reprinted with permission from Burroughs Wellcome Co.)

9. Supplied are 25 mg tab of diethylpropion hydrochloride. Were the physician to order 0.025 Gm po tid ac, how many tab would be administered per dose?

10. Prazepam is supplied in 10 mg scored tab. If the physician orders 15 mg po hs, how many tab should be administered?

11. A client's history indicates that a half tab of phentermine hydrochloride has been taken daily before breakfast. If the medication is supplied in 37.5 mg tab, how many mg have been taken daily?

12. Bromocriptine mesylate tab 1.25 mg are prescribed po bid. How many 2.5 mg scored tab should be administered per dose?

13.   Pentaerythritol tetranitrate 40 mg is prescribed po qid. How many scored 20 mg tab should be administered per dose?

14.   How many gr 1/30 tab of hydromorphone hydrochloride should be administered if gr 1/15 is prescribed?

15.   Carbenicillin indanyl sodium is supplied in tab of 382 mg. If two tab are ordered qid,

a. How many mg should be administered per dose?

b. How many mg should be administered per day?

16. Using the information in Figure 1-2, how many tab should be administered if a half Gm is ordered?

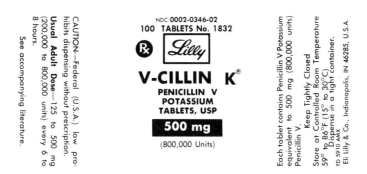

NDC 0002-0346-02
100 TABLETS No. 1832

℞ *Lilly*

V-CILLIN K®

PENICILLIN V
POTASSIUM
TABLETS, USP

500 mg

(800,000 Units)

CAUTION—Federal (U.S.A.) law prohibits dispensing without prescription.
Usual Adult Dose—125 to 500 mg (200,000 to 800,000 units) every 6 to 8 hours.
See accompanying literature.

Each tablet contains Penicillin V Potassium equivalent to 500 mg (800,000 units) Penicillin V. Keep Tightly Closed Store at Controlled Room Temperature 59° to 86°F (15° to 30°C). Dispense in a tight container.
YD 5910 AMX
Eli Lilly & Co., Indianapolis, IN 46285, U.S.A.

FIGURE 1-2 V-Cillin K 500 mg (Reprinted with permission from Eli Lilly and Company)

17. Three tbsp of castor oil are prescribed. On hand is a 150 ml bottle. How many ml should be administered?

18. How many 5 mg cap of prazosin should be administered per dose if 15 mg is to be given daily in three divided doses?

19. A physician's order reads, "Sulindac 100 mg po bid." On hand are scored 200 mg tab of sulindac. How many tab should be administered per dose?

20. The physician orders flurazepam hydrochloride gr s͞s po hs. How many 30 mg cap should be administered?

21. The daily prescribed dosage of gemfibrozil is 1200 mg, half given before breakfast and half before supper. How many 600 mg scored tab should be administered daily?

22. Phenobarbital gr s̅s̅ is ordered po bid. An elixir of 30 mg/7.5 ml is supplied.

    a. How many ml should be administered per dose?

    b. How many tsp?

23. How many 250 mg cap of penicillamine should be administered per dose if 2 Gm are prescribed in four divided doses?

24. Using the information in Figure 1-3, how many scored tab should be administered per dose if the physician orders 30 mg?

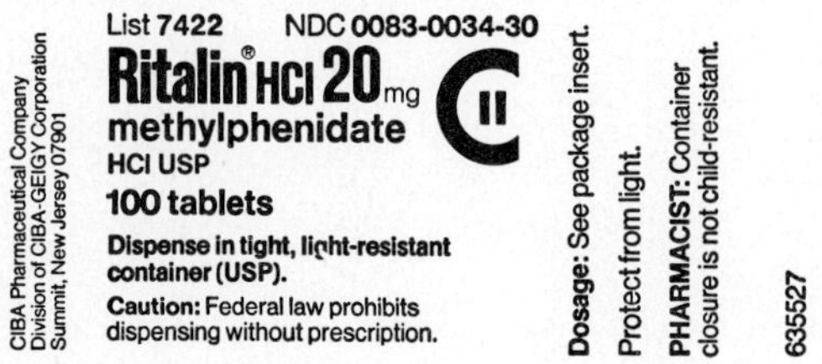

FIGURE 1-3 Ritalin HCl 20 mg (Reprinted with permission from Ciba Pharmaceutical Company)

25. Pentoxifylline is supplied in 400 mg tab. If one tab is ordered twice daily (800 mg/day), how many tab should be administered per dose?

26. Milk of magnesia **℥** ꝥ po hs prn is prescribed. Supplied is a 12 oz bottle of the medication.

 a. How many oz should be administered?

 b. How many tbsp?

 c. How many ml?

27. The physician's order states: "clonidine hydrochloride 0.2 mg po bid." Available on the unit are scored tab of 0.1 mg each. How many tab should be administered per dose?

28. Trimethobenzamide HCl 0.1 Gm is ordered po qid. How many 100 mg cap should be administered per dose?

29. Seventy-five mg of hydroxyzine pamoate is ordered daily in three divided doses. On hand are 25 mg cap. How many cap should be administered per dose?

30. If 200 mg cap of acyclovir have been administered q4h x 5 days,

    a. how many Gm are being administered per dose?

    b. how many Gm are being administered daily?

31. Glyburide 5 mg is ordered po qd with breakfast. Supplied are 2.5 mg scored tab. How many tab should be administered daily?

32. Using the information in Figure 1-4, how many tab should be administered per dose if gr V are ordered po q8h?

For Oral Use Only.

Usual adult dosage — 1 tablet every eight hours.

For complete prescribing information see attached brochure.

Dispense in a tight, light-resistant container as described in USP.

May be taken without regard to meals.

Enteric coated.

Store at controlled room temperature 15° - 30°C (59° - 86° F).

813 966 102

MANUFACTURED BY:
The Upjohn Company
Kalamazoo, Michigan 49001 USA

NDC 0524-0208-01

E-MYCIN®

(erythromycin delayed-release) Tablets, USP

333 mg

100 Tablets

Caution: Federal (USA) law prohibits dispensing without prescription.

Manufactured for:
Boots Pharmaceuticals, Inc.
Shreveport, Louisiana 71106 USA
a subsidiary of
The Boots Company (USA) Inc.

FIGURE 1-4 E-Mycin 333 mg (Reprinted with permission from The Upjohn Company)

33. Tetracycline HCl is available in 500 mg cap. The physician's order reads, "tetracycline HCl 0.5 Gm po qid." How many cap should be administered now?

34. How many 0.4 mg tab of nitroglycerin should be administered if gr 1/150 is ordered?

35. The physician orders benztropine mesylate 1 mg po hs. Available are 0.5 mg tab. How many tab should be administered nightly?

36. Loperamide HCl 1 mg/10 kg body weight is prescribed. Supplied is the liquid formulation of 1 mg/5 ml.

    a. How many mg should be administered to a 44-lb child?

    b. How many ml?

    c. How many tsp?

37. Fenoprofen calcium 0.3 Gm po qid is ordered. On hand are 600 mg scored tab. How many tab should be administered per dose?

38. Lovastatin is supplied in 20 mg tab. How many tab should be administered if 40 mg are ordered po with supper?

39. Twelve hundred mg of tolmetin sodium are ordered in three divided doses. If 400 mg cap are available, how many cap should be administered per dose?

40.   Using the information in Figure 1-5, how many cap should be administered if 0.1 Gm po is ordered nightly?

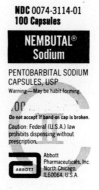

Each capsule contains:
Pentobarbital Sodium
(derivative of barbituric
acid) .... 100 mg
Contains FD&C Yellow No. 5
(tartrazine) as a color additive.
Each capsule bears the ∋ and
Abbo-Code CH for product
identification.
Dispense in a USP tight
container.
See enclosure for prescribing
information.

NDC 0074-3114-01
100 Capsules

NEMBUTAL®
Sodium

PENTOBARBITAL SODIUM
CAPSULES, USP
Warning—May be habit forming

Do not accept if band on cap is broken.
Caution: Federal (U.S.A.) law
prohibits dispensing without
prescription.

Abbott
Pharmaceuticals, Inc.
North Chicago,
IL 60064, U.S.A.

FIGURE 1-5 Nembutal Sodium 100 mg (Reprinted with permission from Abbott Laboratories, Pharmaceutical Products Division)

41.   Atenolol 100 mg po qd is ordered. Supplied is a 100 tab bottle containing 100 mg/tab. How many tab should be administered per dose?

42. Five ml of camphorated opium tincture is prescribed po qid prn. A two-oz bottle is supplied. How many tsp should be administered per dose?

43. The physician orders prochlorperazine 10 mg po q8h x 24 hr. On hand are 5 mg tab. How many tab should be administered per dose?

44. Hydroxyzine hydrochloride is ordered 25 mg po tid. On hand is a one-pint bottle containing 10 mg/tsp.

    a. How many tsp should be administered per dose?

    b. How many ml per dose?

45.   Nitroglycerin tab 0.15 mg sl are ordered q5min x 3. On hand are gr 1/400 tab. How many tab should be administered per dose?

46.   Digoxin is available in scored tab of 0.25 mg (250 mcg). If the prescribed dosage is 0.125 mg po qd, how many tab should be administered?

47.   Terbutaline sulfate 5 mg po is ordered q8h. How many gr should be administered in a 24-hr period?

48. Using the information in Figure 1-6, how many scored tab should be administered if 250 mcg are ordered nightly?

See package insert for complete product information	NDC 0009-0010-01 100 Tablets
Keep container tightly closed	**Halcion**® IV
Dispense in tight, light-resistant container	Tablets triazolam tablets, USP
Store at controlled room temperature 15°-30° C (59°-86° F)	**0.125 mg**
U.S. Patent No. 3,987,052	
812 496 305	**Caution:** Federal law prohibits dispensing without prescription.
The Upjohn Company Kalamazoo, MI 49001, USA	**Upjohn**

FIGURE 1-6 Halcion 0.125 mg (Reprinted with permission from The Upjohn Company)

49. Nystatin oral suspension is ordered one–half million U po q6h. A 60 ml bottle supplies 100,000 U/ml.

a. How many U should be administered per dose?

b. How many ml?

50.   Lactulose syrup is supplied in one-pint bottles containing 10 Gm/15 ml. If 2 tbsp are prescribed qid, how many Gm are delivered per dose?

51.   Terfenadine is available in 60 mg tab. If gr ϯ is ordered po bid, how many tab should be administered per dose?

52.   Two tsp of basic aluminum carbonate gel are prescribed prn. It is supplied in bottles of 12 fluid oz.

a. How many oz should be administered?

b. How many ml?

53. One mg of bumetanide is ordered po qid. How many 0.5 mg tab should be administered per dose?

54. Meclizine HCl is available in 12.5 mg tab. If 25 mg are ordered po qd prn, how many tab should be administered?

55. Using the information in Figure 1-7, how many tsp should be administered if 400,000 U are prescribed?

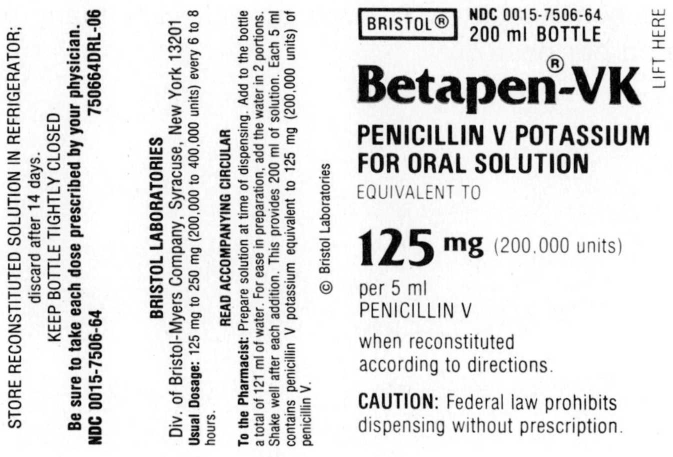

STORE RECONSTITUTED SOLUTION IN REFRIGERATOR;
discard after 14 days.
KEEP BOTTLE TIGHTLY CLOSED
Be sure to take each dose prescribed by your physician.
NDC 0015-7506-64
750664DRL-06

BRISTOL LABORATORIES
Div. of Bristol-Myers Company, Syracuse, New York 13201
Usual Dosage: 125 mg to 250 mg (200,000 to 400,000 units) every 6 to 8 hours.
READ ACCOMPANYING CIRCULAR
To the Pharmacist: Prepare solution at time of dispensing. Add to the bottle a total of 121 ml of water. For ease in preparation, add the water in 2 portions. Shake well after each addition. This provides 200 ml of solution. Each 5 ml contains penicillin V potassium equivalent to 125 mg (200,000 units) of penicillin V.
© Bristol Laboratories

BRISTOL®   NDC 0015-7506-64
200 ml BOTTLE

Betapen®-VK

PENICILLIN V POTASSIUM
FOR ORAL SOLUTION
EQUIVALENT TO

125 mg (200,000 units)

per 5 ml
PENICILLIN V
when reconstituted
according to directions.

CAUTION: Federal law prohibits
dispensing without prescription.

LIFT HERE

FIGURE 1-7 Betapen-VK 125 mg (Reprinted with permission from Bristol-Myers U.S. Pharmaceutical Group)

56. Furosemide 40 mg is prescribed bid. On hand is a 60 ml oral solution containing 10 mg/ml.

a. How many mg should be given per day?

b. How many ml per dose?

57. One hundred mg tab of phenazopyridine hydrochloride are supplied. How many tab should be administered per dose if 200 mg are ordered po tid?

58. The physician's order reads, "Pseudoephedrine hydrochloride gr $\frac{1}{2}$ po qid prn." How many 30 mg tab should be administered?

59. Liothyronine sodium is supplied in 25 mcg tab. How many tab should be administered if 0.025 mg are ordered po qd?

60. How many 1.5 mg scored tab of dexamethasone should be administered if 0.75 mg are prescribed?

61.   Demeclocycline hydrochloride is prescribed for a 75-lb child. If the dosage formulation is 4 mg/lb/day, how many 150 mg tab should be administered per q12h dose?

62.   Piroxicam cap 20 mg po qd are ordered. How many 10 mg cap should be administered daily?

63.   A one oz bottle of ipecac syrup is available. If one tbsp is recommended, how many ml should be administered?

64. Using the information in Figure 1-8, how many cap should be administered per dose if one Gm is ordered po q6h?

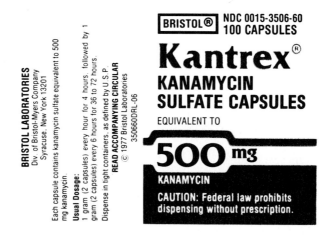

BRISTOL LABORATORIES
Div of Bristol-Myers Company
Syracuse. New York 13201

Each capsule contains kanamycin sulfate equivalent to 500 mg kanamycin.

Usual Dosage:
1 gram (2 capsules) every hour for 4 hours, followed by 1 gram (2 capsules) every 6 hours for 36 to 72 hours.

Dispense in tight containers, as defined by U.S.P.

READ ACCOMPANYING CIRCULAR
© 1977 Bristol Laboratories
350660DRL-06

BRISTOL®   NDC 0015-3506-60
100 CAPSULES

Kantrex®
KANAMYCIN
SULFATE CAPSULES
EQUIVALENT TO

500 mg
KANAMYCIN

CAUTION: Federal law prohibits dispensing without prescription.

FIGURE 1-8 Kantrex 500 mg (Reprinted with permission from Bristol-Myers U.S. Pharmaceutical Group)

65. Nitrofurantoin macrocrystals 50 mg are prescribed po qid.

a. How many gr does this represent per dose?

b. Per day?

66. The physician orders docusate sodium syrup 10 mg po. Available is a 240 ml bottle containing 20 mg/5 ml. How many ml should be administered?

67. Diclofenac sodium 200 mg po is to be given in divided doses qid. If 50 mg tab are supplied, how many tab are to be given per dose?

68. The maintenance dose of sulfisoxazole is 150 mg/kg/24 hr. How many ml should a 29-lb child receive per q6h dose if a 16-oz bottle of the medication supplies a suspension equivalent to 0.5 Gm/tsp?

69. How many 500 mg scored tab of sulfamethizole should be administered per dose if one Gm is prescribed po q6h?

70. Calcitriol is supplied in 0.25 mcg cap. How many cap should be administered if 0.5 mcg are ordered po qd?

71. "RX: megestrol acetate 80 mg po qid." How many scored 40 mg tab should be administered per dose?

72.   Using the information in Figure 1-9, how many ml should be administered per dose to an 88-lb child if the prescribed dosage is 0.15 mg/kg/day in three divided doses?

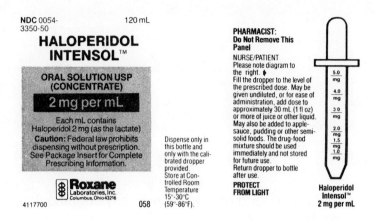

FIGURE 1-9 Haloperidol Intensol 2 mg/ml (Reprinted with permission from Roxane Laboratories, Inc.)

73.   The physician orders reserpine 0.5 mg po qd x 7 days. How many 0.25 mg tab should be administered per dose?

74. Albuterol sulfate syrup is available in 16 oz bottles, 2 mg/5 ml. The physician orders 4 mg po qid.

    a. How many ml should be administered per dose?

    b. How many tsp?

75. Allopurinol is available in scored tab of 100 mg and 300 mg. If the desired dose is 150 mg po qd, how many of which dosage strength would best be given?

76. The usual dosage regimen of erythromycin tab for children is 30–50 mg/kg/day in divided doses.

    a. What is the minimum daily dosage for a 34-kg child?

    b. Maximum daily dosage?

77.   Ranitidine hydrochloride is available in tab of 150 mg each. If the physician orders 0.15 Gm po bid, how many tab should be administered per dose?

78.   After reconstitution with 75 ml of water, a 100 ml bottle of clindamycin palmitate hydrochloride contains 75 mg/5 ml (tsp). How many ml per dose will be required for a 30-kg child if 15 mg/kg/day is prescribed in three divided doses?

79.   How many gr 1/4 thyroid tab should be given if gr 1/2 are prescribed?

80. Using the information in Figure 1-10, how many tab should a 45-kg child receive per dose if the pediatric dosage is 1 mg/lb/day to be given twice daily?

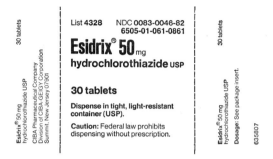

FIGURE 1-10 Esidrix 50 mg (Reprinted with permission from CIBA Pharmaceutical Co.)

81. RX: "nadolol 240 mg po qd." Supplied are scored tab of 120 mg. How many tab should be administered?

82.   Diflunisal is supplied in 250 mg tab. If 0.5 Gm are ordered po q12h prn, how many tab should be administered per dose?

83.   The physician orders 6.25 mg of promethazine HCl po tid. Scored 12.5 mg tab are supplied. How many tab should be administered per dose?

84.   A 16 oz bottle of ferrous sulfate contains 220 mg/5 ml. If one tsp is ordered po tid, how many ml should be administered per dose?

85.   Carisoprodol tab are prescribed 0.35 Gm po tid and hs. How many 350 mg tab should be administered per dose?

86.   Sucralfate is supplied in 1 Gm tab. How many tab should be administered per dose if 1000 mg po qid are ordered?

87.   How many ml of elixir terpin hydrate with codeine should be administered if ℥ ϯ are ordered?

88. Using the information in Figure 1-11, how many tab should be administered if 20 mEq are ordered po daily in two doses?

Dispense in a USP tight container.

Each tablet contains: 750 mg potassium chloride (equivalent to 10 mEq).

Each yellow ovaloid tablet bears the ⊇ and the trademark K-TAB for product identification.

See enclosure for prescribing information.

Filmtab—Film-sealed tablets, Abbott.

©Abbott

Abbott Pharmaceuticals, Inc. North Chicago, IL60064

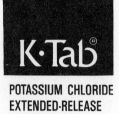

POTASSIUM CHLORIDE
EXTENDED-RELEASE
TABLETS, USP

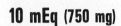

10 mEq (750 mg)

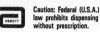

Caution: Federal (U.S.A.) law prohibits dispensing without prescription.

Do not accept if band on cap is broken or missing.

FIGURE 1-11 K•Tab 10 mEq (Reprinted with permission from Abbott Laboratories, Pharmaceutical Products Division)

89. Chlorotrianisene is supplied in 72 mg cap. How many total mg are delivered if one cap is prescribed po bid x 2 days?

90. If the usual starting dosage of albuterol sulfate syrup is 2 mg (1 tsp) po tid to qid, how many ml should be administered per dose if 2 mg/5 ml is available?

91. The physician prescribes promazine hydrochloride 0.2 Gm po q6h. How many 100 mg tab should be administered per dose?

92. Cholestyramine powder is supplied in 9 Gm packets, each containing 4 Gm of anhydrous cholestyramine resin. How many total Gm of the resin does the patient receive if one packet is prescribed po qid?

93.   Baclofen 5 mg po tid x 3 days is prescribed. Ten mg scored tab are available. How many tab should be administered per dose?

94.   Chlorzoxazone is supplied in 500 mg scored cap. If the physician orders 750 mg po qid, how many cap should be administered per dose?

95.   The label on a bottle of aspirin states, "aspirin 5 grains/tablet." How many tab should be administered if 650 mg po are prescribed q4h prn?

96. Using the information in Figure 1-12, how many scored tab should be administered per dose if 0.5 mg are ordered?

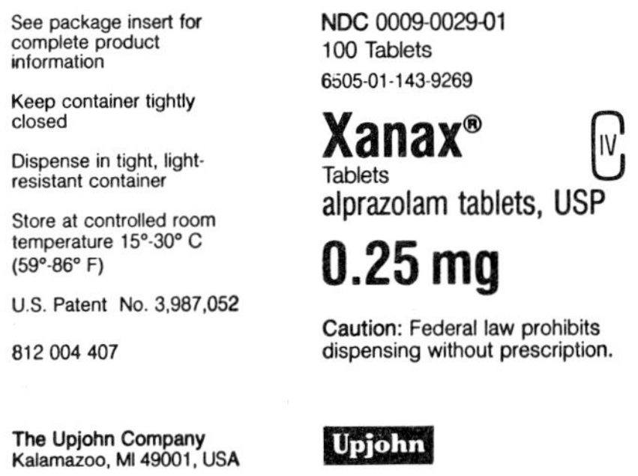

See package insert for complete product information

Keep container tightly closed

Dispense in tight, light-resistant container

Store at controlled room temperature 15°-30° C (59°-86° F)

U.S. Patent No. 3,987,052

812 004 407

NDC 0009-0029-01
100 Tablets
6505-01-143-9269

Xanax®
Tablets
alprazolam tablets, USP

0.25 mg

Caution: Federal law prohibits dispensing without prescription.

The Upjohn Company
Kalamazoo, MI 49001, USA

Upjohn

FIGURE 1-12 Xanax 0.25 mg (Reprinted with permission from The Upjohn Company)

97. The physician orders 0.55 Gm of naproxen sodium po q12h. How many 275 mg tab should be administered per dose?

98. Nortriptyline HCl oral solution is supplied in 16 oz bottles, each 5 ml equivalent to 10 mg base. How many ml should be administered if 30 mg hs are prescribed?

99.   After reconstitution with 75 ml of water, a 100 ml bottle contains 125 mg/5 ml of bacampicillin HCl suspension. How many ml should be administered if 400 mg are prescribed?

100.   Using the information in Figure 1-13, how many tab should be administered if gr s̄s̄ are desired?

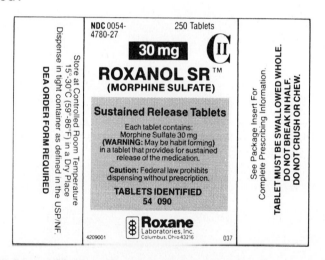

FIGURE 1-13 Roxanol SR 30 mg (Reprinted with permission from Roxane Laboratories, Inc.)

101. Each 480 ml bottle of amantadine hydrochloride syrup contains 50 mg/5 ml. How many ml per dose should be administered if 100 mg are ordered po bid?

102. How many 2 mg scored tab of melphalan should be administered if 6 mg po qd are ordered?

103. If 0.25 Gm of dicloxacillin sodium are prescribed po q6h, how many 250 mg cap should be administered per dose?

104.   Each tab of a calcium supplement contains 500 mg of elemental calcium. How many Gm of calcium are supplied if 3 tab are prescribed daily?

105.   Methyldopa oral suspension is supplied in bottles of 473 ml. Each 5 ml contains 250 mg. If 250 mg po qid are prescribed, how many ml should be administered per dose?

106.   Oxazepam 60 mg po is ordered in four divided doses. How many 15 mg cap should be administered per dose?

107. How many 500 mg cap of hydroxyurea should be administered to a 110 lb patient if the dosage formulation is 20 mg/kg qd?

108. One hundred mg of meclofenamate sodium are ordered po tid. How many Gm should be administered per dose?

109. Propanolol hydrochloride 240 mg po is ordered in three divided doses.

    a. How many 80 mg tab should be administered per dose?

    b. Per day?

110.   Using the information in Figure 1-14, how many scored tab should be administered if 100 mg are prescribed daily, given in two divided doses?

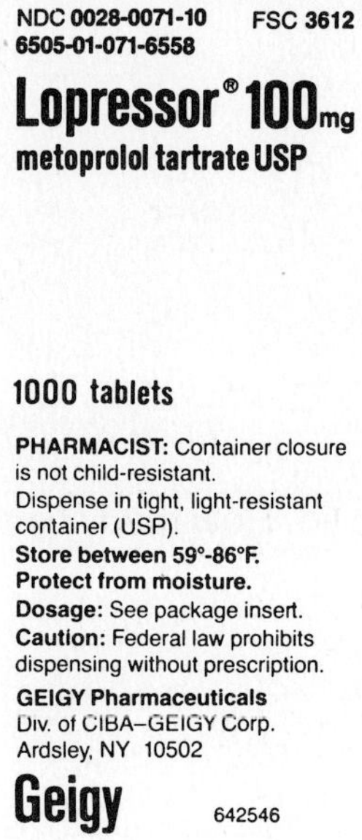

NDC 0028-0071-10   FSC 3612
6505-01-071-6558

Lopressor® 100mg
metoprolol tartrate USP

1000 tablets

PHARMACIST: Container closure is not child-resistant.
Dispense in tight, light-resistant container (USP).
Store between 59°-86°F.
Protect from moisture.
Dosage: See package insert.
Caution: Federal law prohibits dispensing without prescription.
GEIGY Pharmaceuticals
Div. of CIBA-GEIGY Corp.
Ardsley, NY 10502

Geigy   642546

FIGURE 1-14 Lopressor 100 mg (Reprinted with permission from CIBA Pharmaceutical Co.)

111.   A 60 ml bottle of doxycycline monohydrate suspension contains 25 mg/5 ml. If 100 mg are prescribed po q12h,

a. How many mg should be administered per dose?

b. How many ml?

c. How many tsp?

112. Cephradine is available in cap of 500 mg each. How many cap should be administered per dose if one Gm is ordered po q12h?

113. Zidovudine is supplied in 100 mg cap. If 0.2 Gm are prescribed po q4h around the clock,

    a. How many cap should be administered per dose?

    b. How many mg are delivered in a 24-hr period?

114. Each 4 oz bottle of promethazine HCl contains 6.25 mg/5 ml. How many tsp should be administered if 25 mg are prescribed?

115.   If 0.8 Gm of niacin is prescribed po tid, how many 400 mg cap should be administered per dose?

116.   Temazepam is supplied in cap of 15 mg each. How many cap should be administered if gr $\overline{ss}$ are ordered po hs?

117.   A physician's order reads, ". . . doxycycline hyclate 100 mg q12h today, then 100 mg qd.''

       a. How many 100 mg cap should be given on day one?

       b. Thereafter?

118. Buspirone hydrochloride is available in scored tab of 5 mg and 10 mg. How many of which dosage form(s) should be administered per dose if 15 mg tid are ordered?

119. Phenobarbital is available in 30 mg tab.

    a. How many tab should be administered if 0.06 Gm po are ordered?

    b. How many gr does this represent?

120. Using the information in Figure 1-15, how many ml per dose should be administered to a 44-lb child if the pediatric dosage calculation is 40 mg/kg/day, tid?

150 mL CECLOR® CEFACLOR FOR ORAL SUSPENSION, USP

250 mg per 5 mL. Oversize bottle provides extra space for shaking. Store in a refrigerator. May be kept for 14 days without significant loss of potency. Keep Tightly Closed. Discard unused portion after 14 days.

SHAKE WELL BEFORE USING

Usual Dose—Children, 20 mg per kg a day (40 mg per kg in otitis media) in three divided doses. Adults, 250 mg three times a day. See literature for complete dosage information.

Contains Cefaclor Monohydrate equivalent to 7.5 g Cefaclor in a dry pleasantly flavored mixture.

Prior to Mixing: Store at Controlled Room Temperature 59° to 86°F (15° to 30°C)

Directions for Mixing—Add 90 mL of water in two portions to the dry mixture in the bottle. Shake well after each addition.

Each 5 mL (Approx. one teaspoonful) will then contain: Cefaclor Monohydrate equivalent to 250 mg Cefaclor.

Mfd. by Eli Lilly Industries, Inc., Carolina, Puerto Rico 00630 WW 6481 AMX a subsidiary of Eli Lilly & Co., Indianapolis, IN, U.S.A.

NDC 0002-5058-68
150 mL (When Mixed) **M-5058**

℞ *Lilly*

CECLOR®

CEFACLOR FOR ORAL SUSPENSION, USP

250 mg
per 5 mL

CAUTION—Federal (U.S.A.) law prohibits dispensing without prescription.

FIGURE 1-15 Ceclor 250 mg/5 ml (Reprinted with permission from Eli Lilly and Company)

121.   How many 250 mg cap should be administered if mefenamic acid is ordered gr VIIss po stat?

122.   A 5 oz bottle contains 150 ml of an antacid. If ℥ ⅲ are ordered po between meals and hs, how many ml should be administered per dose?

123.   The usual children's dosage of meperidine hydrochloride is between 0.5 mg/lb and 0.8 mg/lb q3–4h prn, dosage not to exceed adult's.

   a. What is the minimum dosage for a 60-lb child?

   b. The maximum dosage?

124. How many ml of mineral oil should be administered if

      a. ℥ ss are ordered po hs?

      b. How many tbsp?

      c. How many oz?

125. The physician orders amoxicillin as the trihydrate, 3 Gm stat as a single oral dose. Supplied are 500 mg cap. How many mg should be administered?

126.   Methocarbamol is supplied in 750 mg tab. How many Gm does the patient receive per dose if two tab are prescribed po qid?

127.   Scored 200 mg tab of carbamazepine are available. If 0.4 Gm are ordered po q12h, how many tab should be given per dose?

128.   The suggested maintenance dosage of sustained release procainamide hydrochloride is 50 mg/kg qd in four equally divided doses.

   a. How many 500 mg tab should a 176-lb patient receive per dose?

   b. Per day?

129. Using the information in Figure 1-16, how many tab should be administered per dose if 3200 mg are to be given daily in four divided doses?

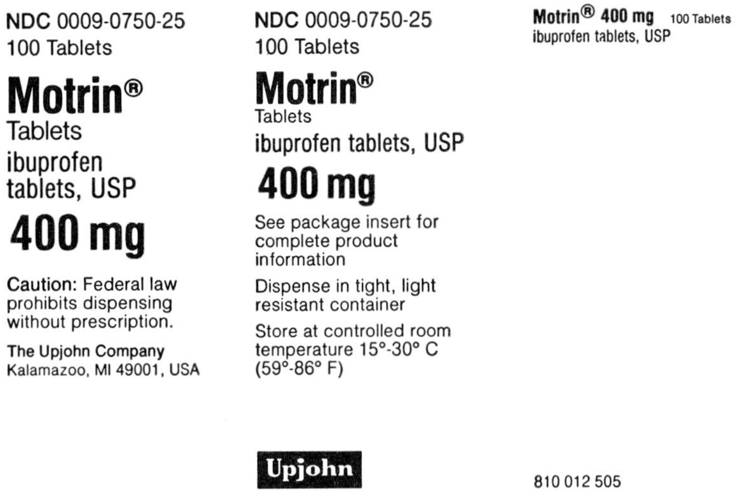

NDC 0009-0750-25
100 Tablets

Motrin®
Tablets
ibuprofen
tablets, USP

400 mg

Caution: Federal law
prohibits dispensing
without prescription.

The Upjohn Company
Kalamazoo, MI 49001, USA

NDC 0009-0750-25
100 Tablets

Motrin®
Tablets
ibuprofen tablets, USP

400 mg

See package insert for
complete product
information

Dispense in tight, light
resistant container

Store at controlled room
temperature 15°-30° C
(59°-86° F)

Motrin® 400 mg   100 Tablets
ibuprofen tablets, USP

Upjohn

810 012 505

FIGURE 1-16 Motrin 400 mg (Reprinted with permission from The Upjohn Company)

130. Folic acid is supplied in 1 mg scored tab. How many tab should be administered if 1000 mcg are prescribed po qd?

131.   Ketoprofen is supplied in 50 mg cap. How many cap should be administered per dose if 0.2 Gm po are ordered daily in four divided doses?

132.   If 0.15 Gm of doxepin HCl are ordered po hs, how many 75 mg cap should be administered?

133.   The dosage for valproic acid is based on the calculation 15 mg/kg/day. How many 250 mg cap should a 70-kg man be given in a 24-hr period?

134. Two hundred mg of diphenhydramine hydrochloride is prescribed po in four divided doses. If 50 mg cap are available, how many should be administered per dose?

135. Nylidrin HCl is supplied in scored 12 mg (gr 1/5) tab. How many tab should be administered if gr 1/10 are ordered?

136. Using the information in Figure 1-17, how many tab should be administered if 0.08 Gm are ordered stat?

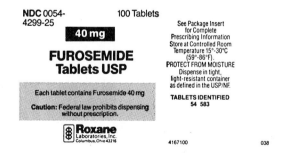

FIGURE 1-17 Furosemide 40 mg (Reprinted with permission from Roxane Laboratories, Inc.)

137.   A 400 mg bottle of famotidine for oral suspension contains, after constitution with
       46 ml of purified water, 40 mg/5 ml. How many ml should be administered if 40
       mg are ordered po hs?

138.   The physician orders 320 mg of acetominophen po q4h prn for a 7-year-old child
       weighing 25 kg. Dosage is based on age and body weight: 6-8 years, 48-59 lb, 2
       tsp. On hand is the liquid medication, 80 mg/1/2 tsp.

       a. How many tsp should be administered per dose?

       b. How many ml?

139.   Butabarbital sodium gr/s̄s̄ is prescribed po hs. If a one-pint bottle contains 30
       mg/5 ml of the elixir, how many ml should be administered?

140. Digitoxin is supplied in scored 0.1 mg tab. How many tab will be required per dose if 0.2 mg po bid x 4 days is prescribed?

141. Medroxyprogesterone acetate is availale in 5 mg scored tab. If 7.5 mg are ordered po qd x 10 days, how many tab should be administered daily?

142. Nafcillin sodium is available in scored 500 mg tab. If 1 Gm is prescribed po q6h, how many tab should be administered per dose?

143. "RX: Iodinated glycerol gr $\frac{1}{2}$ qid with liquid." Supplied are scored 30 mg tab. How many tab should be administered per dose?

144.   Lithium carbonate is supplied in 300 mg tab. If 1200 mg are prescribed po in two divided doses daily, how many tab should be administered per dose?

145.   Using the information in Figure 1-18,

   a. How many mg should be administered per dose if 0.2 Gm po q12h are ordered?

   b. How many ml?

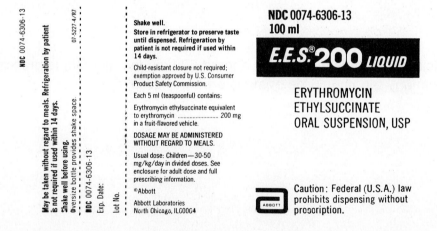

NDC 0074-6306-13

07-5227-4/R7

May be taken without regard to meals. Refrigeration by patient is not required if used within 14 days.

Shake well before using.

Oversize bottle provides shake space.

NDC 0074-6306-13

Exp. Date:

Lot No.

Shake well.

Store in refrigerator to preserve taste until dispensed. Refrigeration by patient is not required if used within 14 days.

Child-resistant closure not required; exemption approved by U.S. Consumer Product Safety Commission.

Each 5 ml (teaspoonful) contains:

Erythromycin ethylsuccinate equivalent to erythromycin .... 200 mg in a fruit-flavored vehicle.

DOSAGE MAY BE ADMINISTERED WITHOUT REGARD TO MEALS.

Usual dose: Children—30-50 mg/kg/day in divided doses. See enclosure for adult dose and full prescribing information.

©Abbott

Abbott Laboratories
North Chicago, ILG00G4

NDC 0074-6306-13
100 ml

E.E.S.®**200** *LIQUID*

ERYTHROMYCIN
ETHYLSUCCINATE
ORAL SUSPENSION, USP

ABBOTT

Caution: Federal (U.S.A.) law prohibits dispensing without prescription.

FIGURE 1-18 E.E.S. 200 liquid (Reprinted with permission from Abbott Laboratories, Pharmaceutical Products Division)

146. Levothyroxine sodium is available in 75 mcg tab. How many tab should be administered if 0.15 mg po is ordered?

147. The physician orders tetracycline hydrochloride 1.5 Gm po stat, then 0.5 Gm q6h x 15 doses.

    a. How many 500 mg tab should be given immediately?

    b. How many per dose, thereafter?

148. The recommended initial pediatric dosage of phenytoin is 5 mg/kg/day in 2–3 equally divided doses. Fifty mg po bid has been ordered for a 44-lb child.

    a. Is this dosage within the recommended guidelines?

    b. How many tab should be administered per dose if 50 mg scored, chewable tab are supplied?

149.   Lorazepam is available in 2 mg scored tab. The order reads 3 mg po tid. How many tab should be administered per dose?

150.   Neomycin sulfate is supplied in 500 mg tab. How many tab should be administered per dose to a 154-lb man if dosage is based on the following: 88 mg/kg/day (q4h x 48 hrs)?

151.   One hundred mg of dipyridamole are ordered po qid. How many 50 mg tab should be administered per dose?

152. One-tenth of a Gm of labetalol hydrochloride is ordered bid. Supplied are 100 mg tab.

    a. How many mg should be administered per dose?

    b. How many tab?

153. A 237 ml bottle of cimetidine HCl contains 300 mg/5 ml. How many ml should be administered per dose if 0.3 Gm are ordered tid with meals and hs?

154. Chloramphenicol is supplied in 250 mg cap. If the recommended dosage is 50 mg/kg/day in 4 equally divided doses, how many cap should a 130-lb patient receive per dose?

155. Using the information in Figure 1-19, how many cap would be required per dose if gr $\dotplus$ po q4h were prescribed?

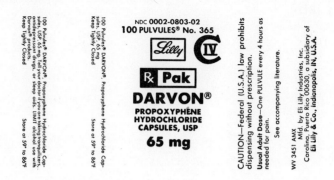

FIGURE 1-19 Darvon 65 mg (Reprinted with permission from Eli Lilly and Company)

156. One Gm of cefadroxil monohydrate is ordered po qd x 10 days. On hand is a 100 ml bottle oral suspension containing 500 mg/5 ml.

   a. How many mg should be administered daily?

   b. How many ml?

157. Chlorpheniramine maleate 4 mg po is ordered q4–6h prn. How many gr does this represent?

158. Potassium chloride is supplied in 750 mg tab, the equivalent, the label states, of 10 mEq. How many tab should be administered per dose if 20 mEq are ordered po bid?

159. The initial dose of trazodone hydrochloride is usually 150 mg/day in divided doses. How many scored 50 mg tab should be administered per day?

160. Chlorpropamide 125 mg po is prescribed qAM with breakfast. On hand are scored 100 mg and 250 mg tab. How many of which dosage form(s) should best be administered?

161. Using the information in Figure 1-20, how many ml should be administered per dose if one Gm is prescribed in two divided doses?

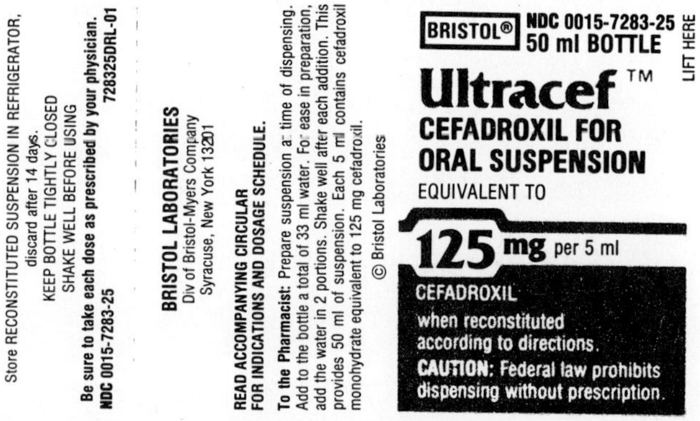

FIGURE 1-20 Ultracef 125 mg/5 ml (Reprinted with permission from Bristol-Myers U.S. Pharmaceutical Group)

162. Dextroamphetamine sulfate is available in 10 mg spansule cap. How many cap should be administered if gr 1/6 po is ordered qAM?

163. Dicyclomine HCl 40 mg is prescribed po q6h. How many 20 mg tab should be administered per dose?

164. The physician orders ethinyl estradiol 50 mcg po bid x 2 wk. The drug is supplied in 0.05 mg and 0.5 mg tab. How many of which dosage strength should be administered per dose?

165. Gemfibozil 1200 mg is prescribed in two divided po ac doses. Supplied are 600 mg scored tab. How many tab should be administered per dose?

166. Crystalline warfarin sodium is available in dosages of 5 mg/scored tab. How many tab should be administered if 7.5 mg are ordered po qd?

167. The physician orders indapamide 5 mg po qd. How many 2.5 mg tab should be administered?

168. Using the information in Figure 1-21, how many scored tab should be administered per dose if 7.5 mg po bid are ordered?

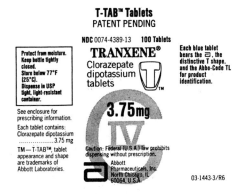

FIGURE 1-21 Tranxene 3.75 mg (Reprinted with permission from Abbott Laboratories, Pharmaceutical Products Division)

169. Diltiazem HCl is supplied in 120 mg scored tab.

a. How many tab should be administered per dose if 60 mg are prescribed po tid?

b. How many gr does this represent?

170.   The physician's order states, "magaldrate antacid ℥ ss between meals and hs." The suspension is supplied in 12 oz bottles (355 ml). How many oz should be administered per dose?

171.   If 5 mg of enalapril maleate are ordered po qd, how many scored 2.5 mg tab should be administered?

172.   Dexchlorpheniramine maleate syrup contains 2 mg/5 ml. How many ml should be administered per dose to a child if 0.5 mg is prescribed po q4–6h prn?

173. Meprobamate is supplied in 400 mg scored tab. If 1.6 Gm are prescribed in four divided doses, how many tab should be administered per dose?

174. Using the information in Figure 1-22, how many tab should be administered per dose if 0.125 mg is ordered po qd?

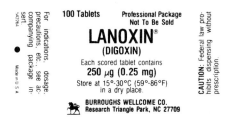

FIGURE 1-22 Lanoxin 250 mcg/tablet (Reprinted with permission from Burroughs Wellcome Co.)

175.   Cephalexin 0.5 Gm po q12h is ordered. Available are 500 mg tab. How many tab should be administered per dose?

176.   Nylidrin HCl 6 mg is prescribed po qid. How many scored 3 mg tab should be administered per dose?

177.   A physician's order states, "Naproxen suspension po 750 mg stat, then 250 mg q8h." Supplied is a 474 ml bottle containing 125 mg/5 ml.

   a. How many ml should be given for the stat dose?

   b. How many ml per dose, thereafter?

178. Captopril is available in tab of 12.5 mg, each with a partial bisect bar. How many tab should be administered per dose if 25 mg are ordered po tid?

179. Scored 50 mg tab of azathioprine are supplied. Using the formulation 1 mg/kg/day in a single dose, how many tab should be administered to a 165-lb patient?

180. Using the information in Figure 1-23, how many tab should be administered if 10 mg (gr 1/6) are prescribed?

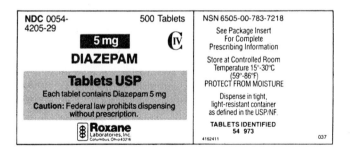

FIGURE 1-23 Diazepam 5 mg (Reprinted with permission from Roxane Laboratories, Inc.)

181. Rescinnamine is supplied in 0.5 mg scored tab. How many tab should be administered per dose if 0.25 mg po qd are ordered?

182. Aluminum hydroxide is supplied in tab of 0.3 Gm (gr V).

    a. If gr X are ordered po between meals and at bedtime, how many tab should be administered per dose?

    b. If tab cannot be tolerated, how many ml of the suspension dosage 325 mg/5 cc can be substituted?

183. Disulfiram is available in scored 250 mg tab. How many tab should be administered if 125 mg po qd are prescribed?

184. How many 0.25 Gm tab of glutethimide should be administered if 500 mg po are prescribed hs?

185. If the prescribed dosage of cephalexin hydrochloride is 4 Gm in four divided doses, how many 500 mg tab should be administered per dose?

186. Colchicine tab are available in a strength of 0.6 mg/tab. If 1.2 mg are ordered po stat, how many tab should be administered?

187. One hundred mg of nitrofurantoin macrocrystals are ordered po qid.

      a. How many Gm are to be given in a 24-hr period?

      b. How many 50 mg cap should be given per dose?

188. Levorphanol tartrate 3 mg is prescribed po q6–8h prn. How many scored 2 mg tab should be administered per dose?

189. Chlorpropamide is supplied in scored tab of 250 mg each. If 125 mg are ordered daily with breakfast, how many tab should be administered?

190. Using the information in Figure 1-24, how many tab should be administered per dose if 2 mg are ordered po q4–6h prn?

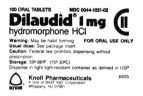

FIGURE 1-24 Dilaudid 1 mg (Reprinted with permission from Knoll Pharmaceuticals)

191. The physician orders naproxen sodium 275 mg po, 2 tab in the morning and 1 tab q6–8h prn. Supplied are 275 mg tab.

    a. How many mg should be administered each morning?

    b. How many mg, per dose, thereafter?

192.   Temazepam is supplied in 15 mg cap.

    a. How many cap should be administered if 30 mg are prescribed po hs?

    b. This latter amount represents how many gr?

193.   Twenty mg of bethanechol chloride are prescribed po qid. If scored 10 mg tab are available, how many tab should be administered per dose?

194.   Ethchlorvynol contains 500 mg per cap. How many cap should be administered if 0.5 Gm are prescribed po hs?

195.   One hundred mg of thioridazine hydrochloride is ordered po in four divided doses. Supplied are 25 mg tab. How many tab should be administered per dose?

196.   If 40 mg of fluoxetine hydrochloride are ordered po bid, how many 20 mg pulvules should be administered per dose?

197.   Desipramine hydrochloride is supplied in 75 mg tab. If 150 mg are ordered po qd, how many tab should be administered in a 24-hr period?

198.   Using the information in Figure 1-25, how many ml per dose should be administered to a 40-lb child if pediatric dosage is based on the formulation 20 mg/kg/day in 3 divided doses?

NDC 0002-5057-18
75 mL (When Mixed) M-5057

℞   *Lilly*

CECLOR®
CEFACLOR FOR
ORAL SUSPENSION
USP

125 mg
per 5 mL

CAUTION—Federal (U.S.A.)
law prohibits dispensing
without prescription.

Usual Dose—Children, 20 mg per kg a day (40 mg per kg in otitis media) in three divided doses. Adults, 250 mg three times a day. See literature for complete dosage information.
Contains Cefaclor Monohydrate equivalent to 1.875 g Cefaclor in a dry pleasantly flavored mixture.
Prior to Mixing, Store at Controlled Room Temperature 59° to 86°F (15° to 30°C).
Directions for Mixing—Add 45 ml of water in two portions to the dry mixture in the bottle. Shake well after each addition.
Each 5 mL (Approx. one teaspoonful) will then contain:
Cefaclor Monohydrate equivalent to 125 mg Cefaclor.
WV 6990 AMX

Mfd. by Eli Lilly Industries, Inc.
Carolina, Puerto Rico 00630, a subsidiary of
Eli Lilly & Co., Indianapolis, IN, U.S.A.

75 mL CECLOR® CEFACLOR FOR ORAL SUSPENSION, USP
125 mg per 5 mL. Oversize bottle provides extra space for shaking. Store in a refrigerator. May be kept for 14 days without significant loss of potency. Keep Tightly Closed. Discard unused portion after 14 days. SHAKE WELL BEFORE USING

FIGURE 1-25 Ceclor 125 mg/5 ml (Reprinted with permission from Eli Lilly and Company)

199.   The usual adult dosage of extra strength buffered aspirin is 2 tab po q4h prn, not to exceed 8 tab daily. If each tab contains 500 mg of the active ingredient, how many mg are in the usual dose?

200.   Five hundred mg of tetracycline are ordered po q12h. How many gr does this represent per dose?

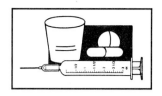

Chapter 2 PARENTERAL MEDICATIONS

INTRAMUSCULAR (IM)/SUBCUTANEOUS (SC)

1. Using the information in Figure 2-1, what percentage of the vial should be used if 1000 mg is prescribed?

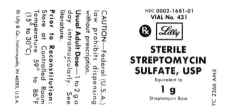

FIGURE 2-1 Streptomycin Sulfate 1 gram (Reprinted with permission from Eli Lilly and Company)

2. If the maintenance dosage of bretylium tosylate is 5 mg/kg q6–8h IM, how many mg per dose should be administered to a 70-kg patient?

3.   Amitriptyline HCl is supplied in 10 ml vials; each vial contains 10 mg/ml. How many ml should be administered per dose if 20 mg IM is prescribed qid?

4.   Dimenhydrinate 50 mg IM is ordered q4h prn. Supplied are 5 ml vials, 50 mg/ml, 250 mg total. How many ml should be administered per dose?

5.   Twenty–five mg of diphenhydramine hydrochloride are ordered IM stat. Supplied is a 1 ml amp containing 50 mg. How many ml should be administered?

6. Tetracycline hydrochloride is available in vials containing 250 mg/2 ml. How many ml should be administered if 0.25 Gm IM are ordered qd?

7. The usual pediatric dosage of meperidine hydrochloride is 0.5 mg/lb to 0.8 mg/lb IM or sc up to the adult dose q3–4h prn.

    a. What is the minimum dosage for a child weighing 90 lb?

    b. What is the maximum dosage?

8. One million, two hundred thousand U of penicillin G benzathine suspension are ordered for deep IM injection. How many ml should be administered if a 2 ml sterile cartridge contains 1,200,000 U?

9. Using the information in Figure 2-2, how many ml should be administered if gr 1 s̄s̄ are ordered?

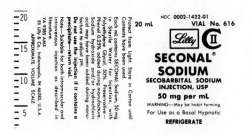

FIGURE 2-2 Seconal Sodium 50 mg/ml (Reprinted with permission from Eli Lilly and Company)

10. Gentamicin sulfate injection is prescribed IM in three equally divided doses, dosage based on the formulation 3 mg/kg/day. How many ml should be administered per dose to a 110-lb patient if a vial contains 40 mg/ml?

11. One Gm of cephazolin sodium injection is ordered IM one hour prior to surgery. After reconstitution with 2.5 ml of diluent, a 1 Gm vial contains 330 mg/ml. How many ml should be administered?

12. Vitamin B_{12} is available in vials containing 1000 mcg/ml. How many ml should be administered if 1 mg IM is ordered?

13. Methoxamine hydrochloride injection is supplied in 1 ml amp containing 20 mg. How many ml would render a dose of 15 mg?

14.   The physician's order states, "morphine sulfate gr 1/6 sc q3–4 prn." Available are amp containing 15 mg (gr 1/4)/ml. How many ml should be administered per dose?

15.   A 2 ml amp of orphenadrine citrate injectable contains 60 mg. How many ml should be administered per dose if 60 mg are ordered q12h prn IM?

16.   A 10 ml multidose vial of levorphanol tartrate contains 2 mg/ml. How many ml should be administered per dose if 3 mg sc q8h prn are prescribed?

17. Using the information in Figure 2-3, how many ml should be administered if 0.5 Gm IM are ordered q12h?

```
BRISTOL®   NDC 0015-3502-24          BRISTOL LABORATORIES, Division of Bristol-Myers Company, Syracuse, NY 13221-4755
                                      CONTENTS: Syringe contains Kantrex (kanamycin sulfate), equivalent to 500 mg kanamycin in 2 ml sterile,
Kantrex (R) KANAMYCIN                 aqueous solution—with 0.66% sodium bisulfite added as an antioxidant, and 2.2% sodium citrate as buffer.
                                      Adjusted to pH 4.5 with H2SO4.
SULFATE INJECTION For I.M. or I.V. Use   USUAL ADULT DOSAGE: Intramuscular—7.5mg/Kg of body weight at 12 hour intervals. Do not exceed 1.5
EQUIVALENT TO                         grams daily. SEE ENCLOSED CIRCULAR FOR DIRECTIONS ON PREPARATION, DOSAGE, AND USE.
500 mg Kanamycin Per 2 ml
                                      1¼" NEEDLE X 22 GAUGE    Patient's Name                          Room No.
CAUTION: Federal law prohibits dispensing without prescription.   DISPOSABLE
                                      SYRINGE                  Doctor                                  Patient's Weight
```

FIGURE 2-3 Kantrex 500 mg (Reprinted with permission from Bristol-Myers U.S. Pharmaceutical Group)

18. A 1 ml amp of phytonadione contains 10 mg. How many ml should be administered if 5 mg IM are prescribed?

19. The physician's order reads, "penicillin G potassium 2,000,000 U IM now." After reconstitution with 3 ml of diluent, a 5,000,000 U vial contains 1,000,000 U/ml. How many ml should be administered?

20. Ten ml of lincomycin hydrochloride injection contain 3 Gm. How many ml should be administered if 600 mg are desired?

21. A 1 ml amp of oxymorphone hydrochloride contains 1.5 mg/ml. How many ml should be administered if 0.5 mg IM is prescribed?

22. Hydrochlorides of opium alkaloids gr 1/6 are prescribed sc q4h prn. How many ml should be administered per dose if 20 mg/ml (gr 1/3) is supplied?

23. Hydralazine hydrochloride is prescribed 40 mg IM. Supplied are 1 ml amp containing 20 mg. How many ml should be administered?

24. An amp of menotropins for injection contains, after reconstitution, 75 IU. How many amp are needed to supply 150 IU?

25. Using the information in Figure 2-4, how many ml should be administered per dose if 5,000 U sc are prescribed q8h?

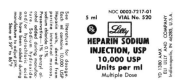

FIGURE 2-4 Heparin Sodium 10,000 USP units/ml (Reprinted with permission from Eli Lilly and Company)

26. If the dosage regimen for bleomycin sulfate is 0.25 to 0.50 U/kg IM,

    a. what is the minimum dosage for a patient weighing 145 lb?

    b. what is the maximum dosage?

27. Prednisolone sodium phosphate injection is supplied in 2 ml vials containing 20 mg/ml. How many m should be administered if 4 mg IM are prescribed?

28. Fifty mg of ranitidine hydrochloride injection are prescribed IM q8h. How many ml should be administered per dose if a 10 ml multidose vial contains 25 mg/ml?

29. The desired dosage of hydromorphone hydrochloride IM is 1 mg. How many m should be administered if 2 mg/ml amp are available?

30. The addition of 2 ml of a specified diluent to a 5 ml dry powder of chlordiazepoxide HCl injectable results in a solution containing 100 mg. How many ml should be administered if 0.1 Gm IM is desired?

31. Twelve and one-half mg of promethazine HCl IM are prescribed q4h prn. How many ml should be administered if amp of 25 mg/ml are available?

32. Butorphanol tartrate gr 1/30 IM is ordered. If 1 ml vials containing 1 mg are available, how many ml should be administered?

33. Using the information in Figure 2-5, how many ml should be administered to a 150-lb patient if the dosage formulation is 0.002 mg/lb?

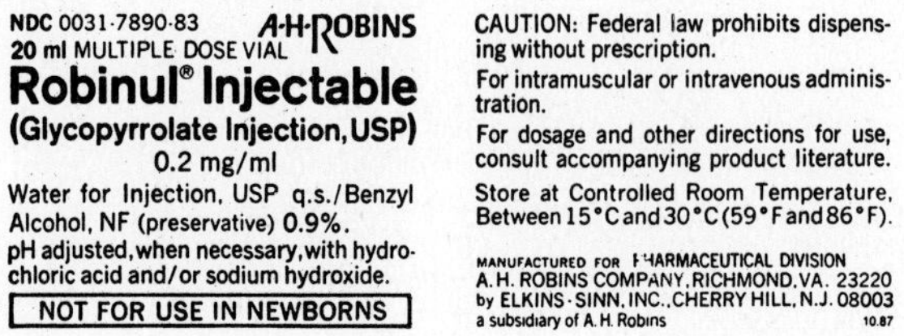

NDC 0031-7890-83   *A·H·ROBINS*
20 ml MULTIPLE DOSE VIAL
Robinul® Injectable
(Glycopyrrolate Injection, USP)
0.2 mg/ml
Water for Injection, USP q.s./Benzyl Alcohol, NF (preservative) 0.9%. pH adjusted, when necessary, with hydrochloric acid and/or sodium hydroxide.

NOT FOR USE IN NEWBORNS

CAUTION: Federal law prohibits dispensing without prescription.
For intramuscular or intravenous administration.
For dosage and other directions for use, consult accompanying product literature.
Store at Controlled Room Temperature, Between 15°C and 30°C (59°F and 86°F).

MANUFACTURED FOR PHARMACEUTICAL DIVISION
A. H. ROBINS COMPANY, RICHMOND, VA. 23220
by ELKINS-SINN, INC., CHERRY HILL, N.J. 08003
a subsidiary of A. H. Robins   10.87

FIGURE 2-5 Robinul 0.2 mg/ml (Reprinted with permission from A. H. Robins Co.)

34. Ceforanide injection 0.5 Gm IM is ordered bid. On hand are vials containing 250 mg/ml. How many ml should be administered per dose?

35. The physician's order reads, "penicillin G procaine suspension 300,000 U deep IM qd." How many ml should be administered if a 1 ml cartridge contains 600,000 U?

36. Isophane insulin is supplied in 10 ml vials; each ml contains 100 U. Indicate how many U should be administered if 40 U sc are ordered daily.

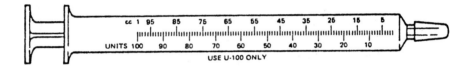

37. Five mg of biperiden lactate are available in each 1 ml amp. If 2 mg IM are prescribed stat, how many ml should be administered?

38.   The physician prescribes 0.05 Gm of benzquinamide hydrochloride IM q4h prn. When reconstituted with 2.2 ml of diluent, each vial contains 50 mg/2 ml. How many ml should be administered?

39.   A 2 ml vial of midazolam HCl injection contains 10 mg (5 mg/ml). How many ml should be administered to a 154-lb patient if a dosage formulation of 0.07 mg/kg is used?

40.   The physician orders phenobarbital sodium gr 1$\overline{ss}$ IM q6h prn. Available is 65 mg/ml. How many ml should be administered?

41. Using the information in Figure 2-6, how many ml should be administered if 0.5 mg is prescribed sc?

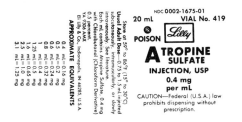

FIGURE 2-6 Atropine Sulfate 0.4 mg/ml (Reprinted with permission from Eli Lilly and Company)

42. A 1 Gm vial of cefoxitin sodium, after an addition of 2 ml of diluent, yields 2.5 ml approximate volume containing 400 mg/ml. If 1000 mg IM is prescribed, how many ml should be administered?

43. Piperacillin sodium 2000 mg IM is ordered. Each 2.5 ml contains 1 Gm of the medication. How many ml should be administered?

44.   The physician's order uses a sliding scale insulin regimen based on ac and hs urinary sugars. Order: isophane insulin suspension 30 U qAM before breakfast; sliding scale for regular insulin:

4 +	20 U
3 +	15 U
2 +	10 U
1 +	5 U

One hr before breakfast, urinary sugar is 3 + . How much of which insulin(s) should be administered?

45.   Dicyclomine hydrochloride is available in a 10 ml vial containing 10 mg/ml. If 80 mg IM are prescribed in four divided doses, how many ml should be administered per dose?

46.   Deslanoside injection is supplied in 2 ml amp. Each 2 ml contains 0.4 mg. How many mg are contained in 8 ml?

47. Naloxone hydrochloride injection 0.2 mg IM is ordered. Supplied is a 10 ml vial containing 0.4 mg/ml. How many ml should be administered?

48. Nalbuphine hydrochloride is ordered 15 mg IM q4h. Supplied are amp containing 10 mg/ml. How many ml should be administered per dose?

49. Using the information in Figure 2-7, how many ml should be administered if 500 mg IM are desired?

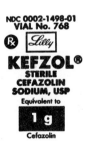

FIGURE 2-7 Kefzol 1 gram (Reprinted with permission from Eli Lilly and Company)

50.   Cyclizine lactate injection is available in amp of 50 mg/ml. If 0.05 Gm IM is ordered q4–6h prn, how many ml should be administered per dose?

51.   Diphylline injection 0.5 Gm is prescribed IM q6h.

    a. If the total of 15 mg/kg q6h should not be exceeded, is this prescription within the recommended guidelines for a 145-lb patient?

    b. If each ml of this medication contains 250 mg, how many ml should be administered per dose?

52.   Terbutaline sulfate 0.25 mg sc is ordered. Supplied are 2 ml amp containing 1 mg/ml. How many ml should be administered?

53. The label on leuprolide acetate injection reads, "1 mg/0.2 ml."

    a. If 1 mg is the recommended dosage, how many doses can be produced from a 2.8 ml multidose vial?

    b. How many m should be administered per recommended dosage?

54. Codeine phosphate injection is available in individual vials containing 60 mg/ml. If gr 3/4 sc is ordered q4h prn, how many ml should be administered per dose?

55. The physician orders penicillin G procaine in aqueous suspension, 1,000,000 U IM daily for ten days. How many ml should be administered if a 10 ml vial contains 3,000,000 U; 300,000 U/ml?

56.   Methylergonovine maleate injection 200 mcg is ordered IM. One ml supplies 0.2 mg. How many ml should be administered?

57.   Using the information in Figure 2-8, how many ml should be administered per dose if 0.5 Gm IM is ordered q12h?

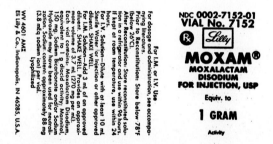

FIGURE 2-8 Moxam 1 gram (Reprinted with permission from Eli Lilly and Company)

58. Calcitonin-salmon injection 100 IU sc qd is prescribed. How many ml should be administered if 2 ml vials contain 200 IU/ml?

59. A 1 Gm size vial of cephradine, after the addition of 4 ml of diluent, yields an approximate volume of 4.5 ml, each ml containing approximately 222 mg. How many ml should be administered if 0.5 Gm IM is prescribed?

60. A 1 Gm vial of streptomycin sulfate contains, after reconstitution with 3.2 ml of water for injection, 250 mg/ml. How many ml should be administered per dose if 0.5 Gm IM is ordered bid?

61. The physician orders regular insulin U–100 sc based on a sliding scale ac and hs
     fingerstick glucose:

Blood Glucose	Insulin Dose in Units
< 150 mg	0
151 – 200 mg	10
201 – 240 mg	15
241 – 280 mg	20
281 – 330 mg	25
> 330 mg	Phone physician

Indicate how many U should be administered if the blood glucose is 239 mg.

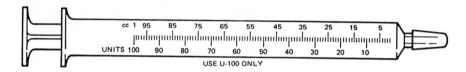

62. Testosterone cypionate injection 200 mg IM is ordered. Supplied are vials containing 100 mg/ml. How many ml should be administered?

63. Fifteen mg of menadiol sodium diphosphate are prescribed IM q12h. How many ml should be administered if a concentration of 10 mg/ml is available?

64. Procainamide hydrochloride injection is supplied in 10 ml vials containing 100 mg/ml. How many ml should be administered if 0.1 Gm IM is ordered?

65. Using the information in Figure 2-9, how many ml should be administered if 40 mg are desired?

NDC 0009-0274-01 5 ml	For IM, intrasynovial and soft tissue injection only. NOT for I.V. use.
Depo-Medrol®	See package insert for complete product information
Sterile Aqueous Suspension	Shake well immediately before using
sterile methylprednisolone acetate suspension, USP	Store at controlled room temperature 15°-30° C (59°-86° F)
	812 152 201
20 mg per ml	The Upjohn Company Kalamazoo, MI 49001, USA

NDC 0009-0274-01 5 ml	For IM, intrasynovial and soft tissue injection only. NOT for I.V. use.
Depo-Medrol®	See package insert for complete product information
Sterile Aqueous Suspension	Shake well immediately before using
sterile methylprednisolone acetate suspension, USP	Store at controlled room temperature 15°-30° C (59°-86° F)
	812 152 201
20 mg per ml	The Upjohn Company Kalamazoo, MI 49001, USA

FIGURE 2-9 Depo-Medrol 20 mg per ml (Reprinted with permission from The Upjohn Company)

66. Furosemide 20 mg IM is ordered. How many ml should be administered if 10 mg/ml are supplied?

67. Hydroxyzine hydrochloride injection is supplied in multidose vials containing 50 mg/ml.

   a. If the dosage formulation for children is 0.5 mg/lb IM, how many mg should a 30-kg child receive?

   b. How many ml?

68. Aztreonam for injection 1,000 mg IM is ordered q12h. How many Gm should be administered per dose?

69. Promazine HCl is supplied in dosage strengths of 50 mg/ml. If 150 mg IM is ordered stat, how many ml should be administered?

70. Heparin sodium injection 8,000 U sc is ordered q8h. Available on the unit are 4 ml vials containing 10,000 U/ml. How many ml should be administered per dose?

71. A 10 ml vial contains 10 mg/ml of metarminol bitartrate. If 4 mg sc are ordered, how many m should be administered?

72.   The physician orders spectinomycin hydrochloride injection 2,000 mg IM. When reconstituted with 3.2 ml of diluent, a 2 Gm vial produces 5 ml of the medication, 400 mg/ml. How many ml should be administered?

73.   Using the information in Figure 2-10, how many ml should be administered if 5 mg IM are ordered?

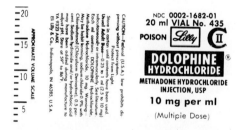

FIGURE 2-10 Dolophine Hydrochloride 10 mg/ml (Reprinted with permission from Eli Lilly and Company)

74. Metoclopramide hydrochloride 10 mg IM is ordered. On hand is a 2 ml single dose vial containing 5 mg/ml. How many ml should be administered?

75. Ethylnorepinephrine hydrochloride is supplied in amp of 2 mg/ml. If 0.1 ml is ordered, how many mg will be delivered?

76. An order for IM lorazepam is derived from the formulation 0.05 mg/kg. How many ml should be administered to a 110-lb patient if 4 mg/ml of the medication is available?

77.   Indicate 27 U of a 100 U insulin.

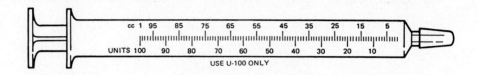

78.   One mg of diazepam IM is ordered. How many ml should be administered if 5 mg/ml is supplied?

79.   How many mg of a solution containing 5 mg/ml will be delivered if 0.5 ml is desired?

80. Dosage strength for IM chlorpromazine is based on the pediatric formulation 1/4 mg/lb of body weight q6–8h prn. How many ml of a 10 ml vial (25 mg/ml) should be administered per dose to a 30-kg patient?

81. Using the information in Figure 2-11, how many ml should be administered if 500 mg are ordered?

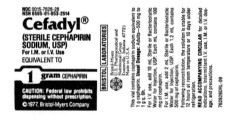

FIGURE 2-11 Cefadyl 1 gram (Reprinted with permission from Bristol-Myers U.S. Pharmaceutical Group)

82. A multiple dose vial of trifluoperazine hydrochloride contains 2 mg/ml. How many ml should be administered per dose if 1.5 mg IM q4h prn are prescribed?

83. If the physician orders 30 mg of methotrexate sodium IM qd x 5 days, how many ml of a 50 mg/2 ml dosage strength would be necessary?

84. A 1500 U vial of hyaluronidase contains, after reconstitution with 10 ml of 0.9% sodium chloride, 150 U/ml. Indicate how many ml should be administered if 75–U sc are ordered stat.

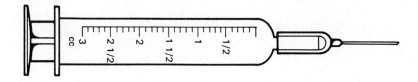

85. Thirty-five U of U–100 insulin are ordered sc ac breakfast. Indicate dosage on illustration.

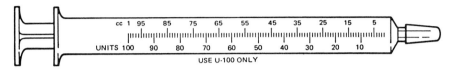

86. Fentanyl citrate injection 0.1 mg IM is ordered. Supplied are amp containing 50 mcg/ml. How many ml should be administered?

87. Three hundred mg of cimetidine hydrochloride injection are ordered IM q8h. How many ml should be administered per dose if vials containing 300 mg/2 ml are available?

88.   Morphine sulfate is available in dosage strengths of 8 mg/ml, 10 mg/ml and 15 mg/ml. How many mg should be administered if gr 1/8 is desired?

89.   The physician orders thiothixene hydrochloride 4 mg IM. After reconstitution with 2.2 ml of water, a vial contains 5 mg/ml of the medication. How many ml should be administered?

90.   Using the information in Figure 2-12, how many U should be administered if 28 U are ordered sc qd before breakfast?

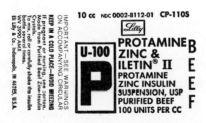

FIGURE 2-12 Protamine Zinc and Iletin II: U–100 insulin (Reprinted with permission from Eli Lilly and Company)

91. Hydroxyzine HCl is supplied in a dosage strength of 25 mg/ml. How many ml should be administered if 0.035 Gm are desired?

92. Bumetanide is supplied in 2 ml amp, containing 0.25 mg/ml. If 0.5 mg IM is ordered qd, how many ml should be administered?

93. Atropine sulfate 0.2 mg contains how many gr?

94. How many ml of 250 mg/ml dosage strength should be administered if 0.5 Gm of dexpanthenol is ordered IM?

95.   If the pediatric dosage formulation of prochlorperazine is 0.06 mg/lb, how many ml of a 5 mg/ml solution should be administered to a 38-kg child?

96.   After reconstitution with 1.8 ml of diluent, a 500 mg vial of ceftriaxone sodium contains 250 mg/ml. How many ml should be administered if 1 Gm is ordered IM in two equally divided doses?

97.   Two and one–half mg of phytonadione are ordered IM. How many m should be administered if a solution of 10 mg/ml is available?

98. The physician orders penicillin G benzathene suspension 900,000 U deep IM. Supplied is a multiple dose vial containing 300,000 U/ml. How many ml should be administered?

99. Using the information in Figure 2-13, how many ml should be administered if 250 mg IM are ordered?

NDC 0002-1497-01
VIAL No. 767

Ⓡ *Lilly*

KEFZOL®

STERILE
CEFAZOLIN
SODIUM, USP

Equiv. to

500 mg

Cefazolin

CAUTION—Federal (U.S.A.) law prohibits dispensing without prescription.
For I.M. or I.V. Use

Dosage—See literature.
To prepare solution add 2 mL Sterile Water for Injection or 0.9% Sodium Chloride Injection. Provides an approximate volume of 2.2 mL (225 mg per mL)
SHAKE WELL   Protect from Light
Prior to Reconstitution: Store at Controlled Room Temperature 59° to 86°F (15° to 30°C)
After Reconstitution: Store in a refrigerator. For Storage Time - See Accompanying Literature. If kept at room temperature, use within 24 hours.
Lyophilized

WV 4520 AMX
Eli Lilly & Co., Indianapolis, IN 46285, U.S.A.

FIGURE 2-13 Kefzol 500 mg (Reprinted with permission from Eli Lilly and Company)

100.   Ergocalciferol in oil suspension is supplied in amp of 12.5 mg (500,000 U)/ml. If 200,000 U IM are ordered qd, how many ml should be administered?

101.   The approximate concentration of ceftizoxime sodium, after reconstitution, is 270 mg/ml. How many ml should be administered per dose if 0.5 Gm IM q12h is ordered?

102.   Hepatitis B Vaccine 0.02 mg is ordered IM. On hand is a 3 ml vial containing 20 mcg/ml. How many ml should be administered?

103. Cefoperazone sodium injection is available in concentrations of 333 mg/ml. How many ml should be administered if 2 Gm IM are ordered in two divided doses?

104. Five thousand U of heparin sodium are ordered sc q12h. Indicate how many ml should be administered if a 4 ml vial contains 10,000 U/ml.

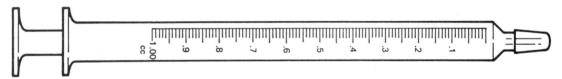

105. Vitamin B_{12} 200 mcg IM is ordered. One oz vials are available and contain 1000 mcg/ml. How many ml should be administered?

106. Three hundred seventy–five mg of hydroxyprogesterone caproate is ordered IM. How many ml should be administered if a multi-dose vial contains 250 mg/ml?

107. If the IM pediatric dosage of fentanyl citrate/droperidol is based on the formulation 0.25 ml/20 lb of body weight, how many ml should a 60-lb child require?

108. Fluphenazine hydrochloride injection is available in 10 ml multi-dose vials containing 2.5 mg/ml. If 1.25 mg IM is ordered, how many ml should be administered?

109. Using the information in Figure 2-14, how many ml should be administered if 3 mg are ordered?

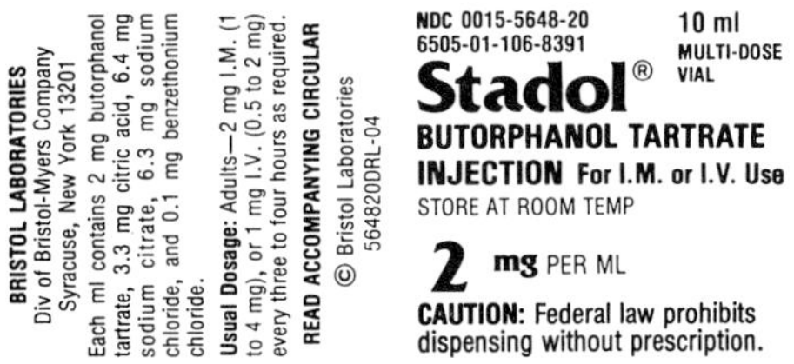

FIGURE 2-14 Stadol 2 mg/ml (Reprinted with permission from Bristol-Myers U.S. Pharmaceutical Group)

110. Each ml of betamethasone sodium phosphate injection contains 4 mg. How many ml should be administered if 2 mg are prescribed?

111. Scopolamine hydrobromide gr 1/120 is ordered. On hand is gr 1/100/ml. How many ml should be administered?

112.   If the dosage for tobramycin sulfate injection is based on the formula 3 mg/kg/day in 3 equally divided doses, how many ml should a 90-kg patient receive per dose if 80 mg/2 ml is supplied?

113.   Vasopressin injection 5 U IM is ordered. On hand is a vial containing 10 U/0.5 ml. How many ml should be administered?

114.   Bethanechol chloride injection is supplied in single dose vials containing 5 mg/ml. How many ml should be administered if 2.5 mg sc are ordered?

115. A 2 Gm vial of cefotaxime sodium injection, after reconstitution with 5 ml of diluent, contains approximately 330 mg/ml. How many ml should be administered if 1000 mg IM are ordered?

116. Pentazocine lactate injection gr 3/4 IM is ordered. Available are amp containing 60 mg/2 ml. How many ml should be administered?

117. The physician's order reads, "trimethobenzamide HCl 0.2 Gm IM qid prn." Each multiple-dose vial contains 100 mg/ml. How many ml should be administered per dose?

118.   Biperiden lactate 2 mg IM is ordered. Ampules containing 5 mg/ml are available. How many ml should be administered?

119.   Using the information in Figure 2-15, how many Gm of the medication will be delivered if one-half vial is administered?

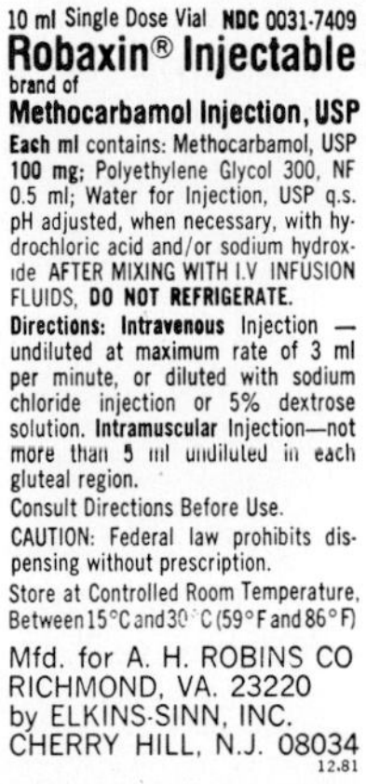

10 ml Single Dose Vial **NDC 0031-7409**
Robaxin® Injectable
brand of
Methocarbamol Injection, USP
Each ml contains: Methocarbamol, USP
100 mg; Polyethylene Glycol 300, NF
0.5 ml; Water for Injection, USP q.s.
pH adjusted, when necessary, with hydrochloric acid and/or sodium hydroxide AFTER MIXING WITH I.V INFUSION
FLUIDS, **DO NOT REFRIGERATE.**
Directions: Intravenous Injection —
undiluted at maximum rate of 3 ml
per minute, or diluted with sodium
chloride injection or 5% dextrose
solution. **Intramuscular** Injection—not
more than 5 ml undiluted in each
gluteal region.
Consult Directions Before Use.
CAUTION: Federal law prohibits dispensing without prescription.
Store at Controlled Room Temperature,
Between 15°C and 30° C (59°F and 86°F)
Mfd. for A. H. ROBINS CO
RICHMOND, VA. 23220
by ELKINS-SINN, INC.
CHERRY HILL, N.J. 08034
12.81

FIGURE 2-15 Robaxin 100 mg/ml (Reprinted
with permission from A. H. Robins Co.)

120.   Buprenorphine hydrochloride injectable is supplied in 1 ml amp containing 0.3 mg each. How many ml should be administered if 0.6 mg are prescribed?

121. Caffeine sodium benzoate 500 mg IM are ordered. On hand is an amp containing 0.5 G/2 ml. How many ml should be administered?

122. Morphine sulfate is supplied in amp containing 15 mg (gr 1/4)/ml. How many ml should be administered per dose if gr 1/8 sc are ordered q4–6h prn?

123. Meperidine hydrochloride 75 mg IM q4h prn is ordered. On hand are cartridges containing 100 mg/ml. How many ml should be administered per dose?

124. Kanamycin sulfate injection is supplied in dosage strengths of 75 mg/2 ml.

a. If the dosage is based on the formulation 15 mg/kg/day in divided doses, how many mg should a 7.7-lb infant receive daily?

b. How many ml should be administered if the medication is ordered q12h?

125. The physician orders dyphylline injection 0.5 Gm IM. How many ml should be administered if 250 mg/ml are available?

126. Hyoscyamine sulfate injection 0.25 mg IM is ordered. A sterile solution containing 0.5 mg/ml is supplied. How many ml should be administered?

127. Dexamethasone sodium phosphate injection is supplied in units of 4 mg/ml. How many ml will be required if 6 mg IM are prescribed?

128. Ten mg of aurothioglucose suspension are ordered by the IM route. If multiple dose vials containing 50 mg/ml are available, how many ml should be administered?

129. Using the information in Figure 2-16, how many ml should be administered if 600,000 U IM are ordered in two divided doses?

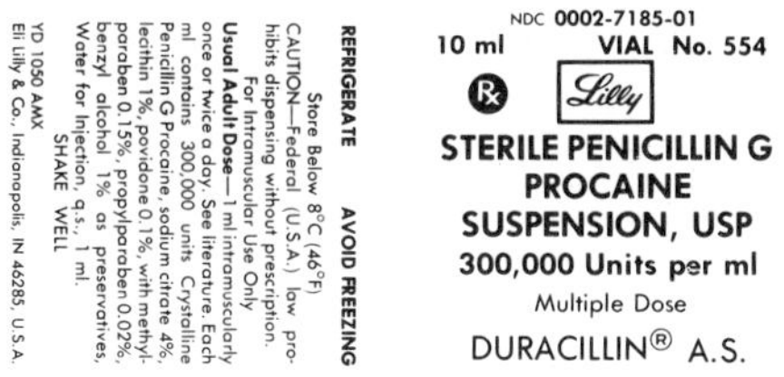

NDC 0002-7185-01

10 ml   **VIAL No. 554**

℞   *Lilly*

**STERILE PENICILLIN G
PROCAINE
SUSPENSION, USP**
300,000 Units per ml
Multiple Dose
DURACILLIN® A.S.

FIGURE 2-16 Penicillin G Procaine 300,000 U/ml (Reprinted with permission from Eli Lilly and Company)

130.   Sixty mg of orphenadrine citrate injectable is ordered IM q12h prn. On hand is a 2 ml amp containing 60 mg. How many ml should be administered per dose?

131.   How many ml of a solution containing 10 mg/ml should be administered if 0.01 Gm edrophonium chloride IM is needed?

132.   Methylprednisolone sodium succinate 80 mg IM is ordered. How many ml should be administered if a vial contains 40 mg/ml?

133.   One ml of pentobarbital sodium contains gr 3/4. How many ml should be administered if gr $\overline{ss}$ are ordered IM?

134. The recommended dose of iron and B complex injectable for children is 0.5 ml IM once a week. How many m should be administered?

135. Using the information in Figure 2-17, how many ml should be administered per dose if 10,000 U sc q8h are prescribed?

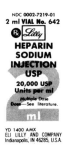

FIGURE 2-17 Heparin Sodium 20,000 U/ml (Reprinted with permission from Eli Lilly and Company)

136. After reconstitution with 2 ml of sterile water, a vial of deferoxamine mesylate contains 250 mg/ml. How many ml should be administered if 0.5 Gm IM are ordered?

137.   Phentolamine mesylate 5 mg is dissolved in 1 ml sterile water for injection. How many ml should be administered if 3 mg IM are ordered as a one-time dose?

138.   Nalbuphine hydrochloride injection is supplied in amp containing 20 mg/ml. How many ml should be administered per dose if 10 mg (gr 1/6) IM are ordered q3–6h prn?

139.   The physician orders dexamethasone acetate suspension injection 12 mg IM. How many ml should be administered if 5 ml multiple-dose vials contain 16 mg/ml?

140. Imipramine hydrochloride is supplied in a dosage strength of 25 mg/2 ml. How many ml should be administered if 25 mg IM is ordered daily in four divided doses?

141. After reconstitution with 1.5 ml diluent, a 500 mg vial of ceftazidime injection yields an approximate volume of 1.8 ml. Each ml contains approximately 280 mg. If 500 mg IM are ordered q8h, how many ml should be administered per dose?

142. Folic acid parenteral solution is supplied in vials containing 5 mg/ml. If 1 mg is ordered IM, how many ml should be administered?

143. Using the information in Figure 2-18, how many ml should be administered per dose to a 143-lb patient if the dosage is based on the formulation 15 mg/kg/day in three equally divided doses?

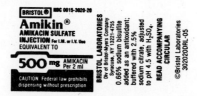

FIGURE 2-18 Amikin 500 mg (Reprinted with permission from Bristol-Myers U.S. Pharmaceutical Group)

144. The physician orders loxapine hydrochloride 12.5 mg IM q6h. How many ml should be administered per dose if the medication is supplied in multi-dose vials containing 50 mg/ml?

145. Dosage for pentamidine isethionate is based on the formulation 4 mg/kg (qd x 14 days). How many Gm would a 154-lb patient require daily?

146.   Benztropine mesylate injection is supplied in dosage strengths of 1 mg/ml. How many ml should be administered if 0.75 mg IM hs are prescribed?

147.   Cortisone acetate is available in vials containing 50 mg/ml. If 20 mg IM are ordered, how many ml should be administered?

148.   Thirty-five mg of gold sodium thiomalate injection IM are ordered. How many ml should be administered if 10 ml vials contain 50 mg/ml?

149.   Using the information in Figure 2-19, how many ml should be administered per dose if 0.25 Gm IM q6h is ordered?

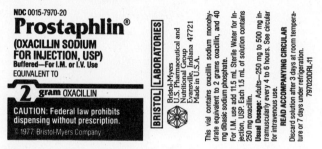

FIGURE 2-19 Prostaphlin 2 grams (Reprinted with permission from Bristol-Myers U.S. Pharmaceutical Group)

150.   Ampules of buprenorphine hydrochloride contain 0.3 mg/ml (gr 1/200/ml). How many ml should be administered if gr 1/100 is desired?

151. A 150 mg vial of colistimethate sodium contains, after reconstitution with 2.0 ml of sterile water, 75 mg/ml. How many ml should a 117-lb patient receive per dose if the dosage is based upon the formulation 2.5 mg/kg/day in four divided doses?

152. The physician orders regular insulin sc ac on a sliding scale based on urinary sugars:

Urinary Sugar	Insulin Dosage in Units
4 +	30
3 +	25
2 +	20
1 +	0

At 11:30 AM, before lunch, urinary sugar is 3 +. How many U should be administered?

153. Meperidine hydrochloride 30 mg IM q4h prn is ordered. On hand is a cartridge containing 50 mg/ml. How many ml should be administered per dose?

154. The physician orders ceftriaxone sodium 0.5 Gm IM q12h. On hand are amp containing 250 mg/ml. How many ml should be administered per dose?

155. Menadiol sodium diphosphate injection is supplied in amp containing 10 mg/ml. How many ml should be administered if 7.5 mg are ordered IM qd?

156. Ampules of chlorprothixene HCl contain 25 mg/2 ml. How many ml should be administered if 10 mg IM are ordered?

157. The dosage strength of netilmicin sulfate injection is based on the formulation 3–4 mg/kg/day. If 100 mg/ml of the medication is available,

    a. what is the minimum daily dosage in ml for a 165-lb patient?

    b. what is the maximum daily dosage in ml for a 165-lb patient?

158. Hyoscyamine sulfate injection is supplied in a 10 ml vial containing 0.5 mg/ml (gr 1/120). How many ml should be administered if gr 1/250 sc are ordered?

159. Using the information in Figure 2-20, how many ml should be administered if 250 mg IM are desired?

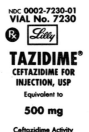

FIGURE 2-20 Tazidime 500 mg (Reprinted with permission from Eli Lilly and Company)

160.   Cefonicid sodium is available in dosage strengths of 325 mg/ml. How many ml should be administered if 0.5 Gm IM are ordered?

Questions 161 — 170: Indicate answers on syringes illustrated.

161.   If the pediatric dosage of penicillin G sodium injection is based on the formulation 25,000 U/kg, how many ml of a 1,000,000 U/ml solution should be administered to a 62-lb patient?

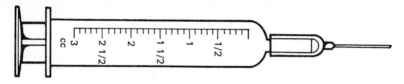

162.   The approximate concentration of a 2 Gm size vial of cefotetan disodium, after reconstitution with 3 ml of diluent, is 471.5 mg/ml. How many ml should be administered if 1 Gm IM is prescribed?

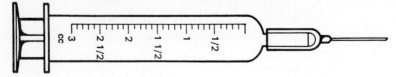

163. Leuprolide acetate injection is supplied in the dosage strength 1 mg/0.2 ml. How many ml should be administered if gr 1/60 sc is desired?

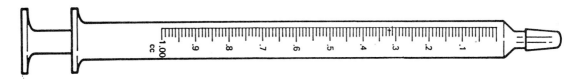

164. Isoproterenol hydrochloride injection 1:5000 is ordered sc 20 mcg. How many ml should be administered if amp containing 0.2 mg/ml are available?

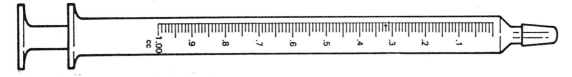

165. Penicillin G benzathine and penicillin G procaine suspension injection is supplied in cartridges of 1.2 million U/2 ml. How many ml should be administered if 600,000 U are ordered?

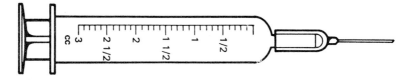

166. The physician orders polyestradiol phosphate 0.04 Gm IM. After reconstitution with 2 ml sterile diluent, an amp contains 40 mg. How many ml should be administered?

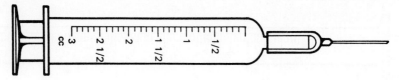

167. Each ml of pentagastrin contains 0.25 mg (250 mcg).

a. What should the dosage for a 70-kg patient be if the dosage formulation 6 mcg/kg is used?

b. How many ml should be administered?

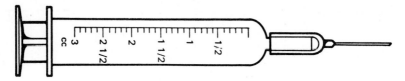

168. Methylprednisolone acetate suspension 40 mg IM is ordered. How many ml should be administered if a dosage strength of 80 mg/ml is available?

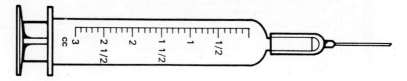

169. Using the information in Figure 2-21, how many ml should be administered if 30 mg IM are desired?

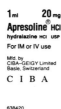

1 ml   20 mg
Apresoline® HCl
hydralazine HCl USP
For IM or IV use

Mfd. by
CIBA–GEIGY Limited
Basle, Switzerland
C I B A

638420

FIGURE 2-21 Apresoline HCl 20 mg/1 ml (Reprinted with permission from CIBA Pharmaceutical Co.)

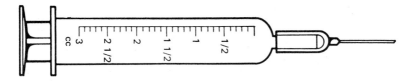

170. Iron dextran is supplied in 10 ml multidose vials containing 50 mg/ml.

   a. How many Gm does this latter value represent?

   b. Indicate how many ml should be administered if 50 mg IM are ordered?

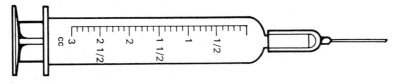

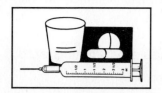

Chapter 3 INTRAVENOUS FLUIDS and MEDICATIONS

GUIDELINES FOR IV ADMINISTRATION

1. The drop rate for IV solutions must be measured in whole numbers. Round to the nearest whole number with 0.5 or more rounded up and 0.4 or less rounded down.

2. IV flow rates may be adjusted up or down to 25% over initial flow rate (policy may dictate a lower percentage of adjustment or no adjustment without an order). Larger increases or decreases in flow rate require physician order.

3. Always use macrodrip if the amount to be infused IV is over 125 ml/hr; use microdrip if the amount to be infused is under 80 ml/hr.

4. Use microdrip for those who need precise amount of fluids, such as infants, children, the critically ill, the elderly, or anyone who needs a more careful monitoring of fluids or drugs.

5. IV medications given one time or intermittently should be diluted in 50–100 ml of fluid to be given over 30–60 minutes as directed in manufacturer's information.

6. When calculating IV total intake, IVPB, volume control chambers or any other infusion device, amounts should be included in the total intake. (Policy may dictate fluid inclusions in intake totals.)

7. All infused IV medications must be ordered in a specified concentration and period of time (when appropriate) to be given in order to assure accurate calculation and administration.

Refer to the IV set shown in Figure 3-1 for problems 1–35.

1. The physician orders an IV infusion of 1 L to be given over 10 hours.

   a. Amount infused/hr?

   b. Drop rate/min?

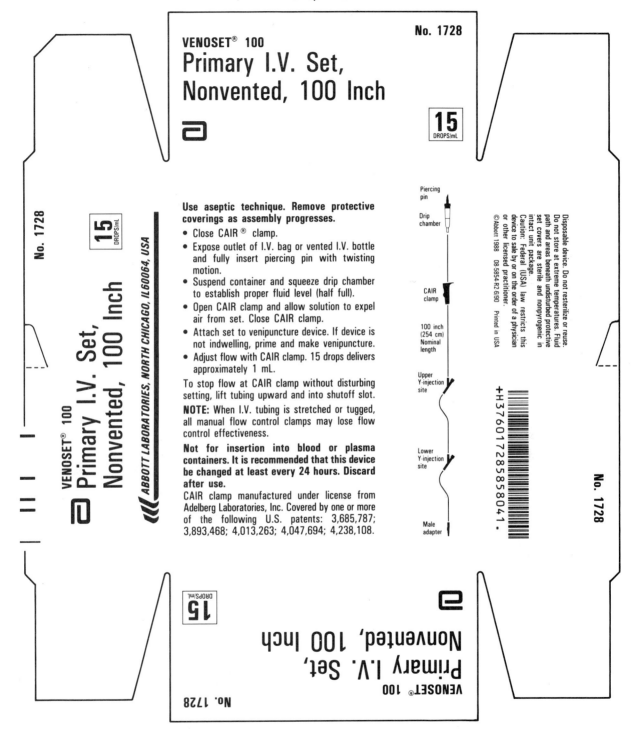

No. 1728

VENOSET® 100

Primary I.V. Set, Nonvented, 100 Inch

15 DROPS/mL

Use aseptic technique. Remove protective coverings as assembly progresses.

- Close CAIR® clamp.
- Expose outlet of I.V. bag or vented I.V. bottle and fully insert piercing pin with twisting motion.
- Suspend container and squeeze drip chamber to establish proper fluid level (half full).
- Open CAIR clamp and allow solution to expel air from set. Close CAIR clamp.
- Attach set to venipuncture device. If device is not indwelling, prime and make venipuncture.
- Adjust flow with CAIR clamp. 15 drops delivers approximately 1 mL.

To stop flow at CAIR clamp without disturbing setting, lift tubing upward and into shutoff slot.

NOTE: When I.V. tubing is stretched or tugged, all manual flow control clamps may lose flow control effectiveness.

Not for insertion into blood or plasma containers. It is recommended that this device be changed at least every 24 hours. Discard after use.

CAIR clamp manufactured under license from Adelberg Laboratories, Inc. Covered by one or more of the following U.S. patents: 3,685,787; 3,893,468; 4,013,263; 4,047,694; 4,238,108.

Piercing pin

Drip chamber

CAIR clamp

100 inch (254 cm) Nominal length

Upper Y-injection site

Lower Y-injection site

Male adapter

Disposable device. Do not resterilize or reuse. Do not store at extreme temperatures. Fluid path and areas beneath undisturbed protective set covers are sterile and nonpyrogenic in intact unit package.
Caution: Federal (USA) law restricts this device to sale by or on the order of a physician or other licensed practitioner.
©Abbott 1988   08-5854-R2-6/90   Printed in USA

ABBOTT LABORATORIES, NORTH CHICAGO, IL 60064, USA

FIGURE 3-1 Nonvented Primary IV Set; 15 drops/ml
(Reprinted with permission from Abbott Laboratories Pharmaceutical Products Division)

2. Three thousand ml of D5 in 0.45% NS is ordered to be given in 24 hours.

    a. Amount infused/hr?

    b. Drop rate/min?

3. A 1 L bottle of D5W is to be infused over 24 hours KVO.

    a. Drop rate/min?

4. An IV infusion of 2 L D5W is to be given in 24 hours.

    a. Amount infused/hr?

    b. Drop rate/min?

5. Five hundred ml is to be infused in 6 hours.

    a. Drop rate/min?

6. The following fluids are to be infused over 18 hours in this order: 1000 ml D5W, 500 ml Ringer's Lactate, 500 ml D5W.

    a. Total amount infused in L?

    b. Drop rate/min?

7. The following solutions are to be infused IV at 120 ml/hr: 1 L D5W, 1 L Ringer's Lactate, 1000 ml D5NS.

    a. Total amount to be infused?

    b. Time it will take to infuse total amount?

    c. Drop rate/min?

8. An infusion is running at 25 gtt/minute.

    a. Amount infused/hr?

    b. Amount infused in 8 hours?

9. Two L of D5W is ordered IV to be infused over 20 hours. After 16 hours, 500 ml remain in the second bottle.

    a. Initial drop rate/min?

    b. Adjusted drop rate/min?

10. The physician's order is to infuse 500 ml/5 hr.

    a. Time it will take to infuse total amount?

    b. Drop rate/min?

11. An infusion of D5W is running at 21 gtt/min?

    a. Amount infused in 5 hours?

12. Three L D5W is ordered to be infused by continuous IV over 24 hours. After 18 hours, 500 ml remain to be infused.

    a. Initial drop rate/min?

    b. Adjusted drop rate/min?

13. An IV infusion of 1500 ml D5W is to be given in 16 hours.

    a. Amount infused/hr?

    b. Drop rate/min?

14. Two L of D5 in 0.45% NS is ordered to be given in 20 hours.

     a. Drop rate/min?

15. One thousand ml of D2.5W is to be infused in 12 hours.

     a. Drop rate/min?

16. A liter of NS is ordered to be given in 10 hours. The IV is started at 10 AM and at 5 PM, 600 ml still remain in the bottle.

     a. Drop rate/min?

     b. Amount infused by 5 PM?

     c. Amount that should have been infused by 5 PM?

     d. Would infusion of the remaining 600 ml in the time left be within the acceptable 25% allowable increase in rate?

17. Two thousand ml of D5W is started at 4 PM at 125 ml/hr.

    a. Completion time for IV?

    b. Drop rate/min?

18. An order states that 500 ml albumin 5% is to be given in 4 hours.

    a. Drop rate/min?

19. Three L of D5W is ordered to be given in 24 hours.

    a. Amount to be infused in 8 hours?

    b. Drop rate/min?

20.   A primary line of 1 L D5W is to be infused in 8 hours.

   a. Drop rate/min?

21.   A combination of IV fluids is ordered to be given in 24 hours as follows: 500 ml D5W, 1000 ml Ringer's Lactate, 1000 ml D5W.

   a. Total amount to be infused in L?

   b. Drop rate/min?

22.   Two liters of D5W is ordered to be given in 18 hours. The IV is started at 8 AM and at 8 PM, 1 L has been infused and 600 ml still remain in the second L.

   a. Amount infused by 8 PM?

   b. Amount that should have been infused by 8 PM?

   c. Initial drop rate/min?

   d. Adjusted drop rate/min to infuse remaining amount?

23. Two thousand ml of D5W is started with orders to complete in 24 hours. In 15 minutes, 50 ml has been infused.

    a. Actual drop rate/min?

    b. Is the amount infused correct?

24. A continuous IV of 1000 ml D5W with 40 mEq potassium chloride (KCl) added is ordered. The IV is discontinued with 700 ml remaining.

    a. Amount of KCl infused in mEq?

    b. Drop rate/min if ordered to infuse in 8 hours?

25. Dextran 40 (10% in D5W) 500 ml IV over 8 hours and repeated doses are ordered to be given for an additional 2 days.

    a. Amount to be infused in ml/hr?

    b. Total amount to be infused in 3 days?

    c. Drop rate/min?

26. Five hundred ml of plasma protein fraction is ordered to be given at 6 ml/min.

a. Amount to be infused/hr?

b. Drop rate/min?

27. An order for heparin sodium 30,000 U/24 hours in 1000 ml NS is to be given by continuous IV infusion.

a. Amount in U/hr?

b. Drop rate/min?

28. Premixed heparin sodium is available in 25,000 U/500 ml for continuous IV infusion.

a. Concentration of solution in U/ml?

The order is to give 1000 U/hr.

b. Infusion rate in ml/hr?

29. Aminophylline is available in 1000 mg/1000 ml for continuous IV infusion.

    a. Concentration of solution in mg/ml?

    The order is to give 20 mg/hr.

    b. Infusion rate in ml/hr?

30. Magnesium sulfate (10%) 4 Gm in 250 ml D5W is prepared for an IV infusion. Orders are to give 2 ml/min.

    a. Amount of solution to be infused in ml/hr?

    b. Drop rate/min?

31. Regular insulin 500 U is added to 500 ml NS with orders to give 10 U/hr IV.

    a. Amount to give in ml/hr?

    b. Drop rate/min?

32.   Heparin sodium 40,000 U is added to 1 L NS. Orders are to administer 20,000 U in 12 hours by continuous IV infusion.

a. Amount of total IV to infuse in ml/12 hr?

b. Amount of drug given in U/hr?

c. Drop rate/min?

33.   Dextran 40, 10 ml/kg is ordered for an adult weighing 58 kg.

a. Amount to be infused?

34.   Lidocaine hydrochloride 0.4% in 500 ml D5W at a concentration of 4 mg/ml is available for IV infusion. An order is written to give 8 mcg/kg/min for an adult weighing 65 kg.

a. Amount of drug in mcg/ml?

b. Amount to give in ml/min?

35. One L of D5W containing 25 mg nitroglycerin for IV infusion is on hand to administer 5 mcg/min dose.

   a. Concentration of solution in mcg/ml?

   b. Flow rate in ml/hr to give 5 mcg/min?

Refer to Figure 3-2 for problems 36–69.

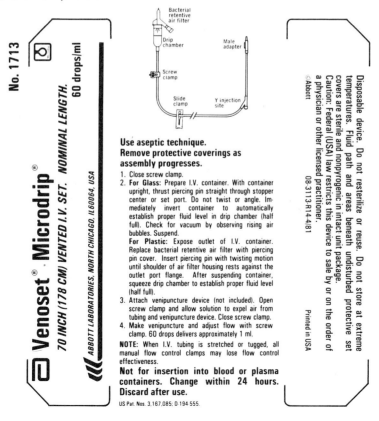

FIGURE 3-2 Venoset Microdrip IV Set; 60 drops/ml
(Reprinted with permission from Abbott Laboratories, Pharmaceutical Products Division)

36. An order for an IV infusion of 1500 ml D5W is to be given in 18 hours.

    a. Amount infused/hr?

    b. Drop rate/min?

37. One L of D5 in 0.45% NS is ordered to be given in 12 hours.

    a. Drop rate/min?

38. Five hundred ml of D2.5W is to be infused in 12 hours.

    a. Amount infused/hr?

    b. Drop rate/min?

39. One L of D5W is ordered to be given over 24 hours KVO.

    a. Drop rate/min?

40. Two hundred fifty ml D5W is to be infused in 4 hours.

    a. Drop rate/min?

41. Nine hundred ml of NS is ordered to run at 75 ml/hr.

    a. Length of time to infuse total amount?

    b. Drop rate/min?

42.   One thousand ml of D5W is running at drop rate/min of 50.

　　　a. Amount infused/hr?

　　　b. Length of time to infuse total amount?

43.   There is an order for an individual to receive 600 ml over 24 hours.

　　　a. Amount infused in ml/hr?

　　　b. Drop rate/min?

44.   An individual has orders to receive D5W at 60 ml/hr.

　　　a. Amount to give in ml for 6 hours?

　　　b. Drop rate/min?

45. Two hundred fifty ml D5W is ordered to be given over 8 hours.

    a. Drop rate/min?

46. An order states that 500 ml is to be infused in 5 hours.

    a. Drop rate/min?

47. Three thousand ml of D5 in 0.45% NS is ordered to be given over 24 hours.

    a. Drop rate/min?

48. The following fluids are to be infused over 24 hours in this order: 1000 ml D5W, 1000 ml Ringer's Lactate, 500 ml D5W.

    a. Total amount infused?

    b. Drop rate/min?

49. An infusion is running at 25 gtt/min.

    a. Amount infused in 6 hours?

50. One L of D5W is started at 8 AM at 100 ml/hr.

    a. Completion time for IV?

    b. Drop rate/min?

51. Morphine sulfate 3 mg/hr IV is ordered to be given. A preparation of 100 mg in 250 ml D5W is ready for infusion.

    a. Amount in mg/ml?

    b. Amount in ml/hr?

    c. Drop rate/min?

52. One L infusion of hetastarch is to be given at 5 ml/kg/hr to an individual weighing 143 lb.

    a. Weight in kg?

    b. Amount in ml/hr?

53. Isoproterenol hydrochloride is to be given IV in a 1:250,000 solution. On hand is a 1:5000/ml solution to be added to a D5W infusion.

    a. Amount of 1:5000/ml solution to be added in ml?

54.   Nitroglycerin is available in 25 mg vials consisting of 5 mg/ml. The vial is diluted in 500 ml D5W for an order to administer 10 mcg/min.

   a. Concentration of solution in mcg/ml?

   b. Flow rate in ml/hr?

   c. Flow rate in drops/min?

55.   Aminophylline 0.5 mg/kg/hr is ordered IV for an individual weighing 132 lb. One L of fluid containing 1000 mg of the drug is hung to administer the medication.

   a. Weight in kg?

   b. Concentration of drug in mg/ml?

   c. Amount to be infused in ml/hr?

   d. Flow rate in drops/min?

56.   Aminophylline 1000 mg/1 L D5W is hung for IV infusion with an order to administer 45 mg/hr.

   a. Concentration of solution in mg/ml?

   b. Infusion rate in ml/hr?

57. An order to infuse 1000 U/hr of heparin sodium is written for an individual. A mixture of 25,000 U/1000 ml 0.45% NS is prepared for administration.

    a. Concentration in U/ml?

    b. Drop rate/min?

58. An order to infuse 500 U/hr of heparin sodium using a pre-mixed container of 25,000 U/500 ml in 0.45% NS.

    a. Concentration in U/ml?

    b. Amount infused in ml/hr?

    c. Amount in ml/hr to increase for each increase of 50 U/hr?

59. One L of D5W contains 10,000 U heparin sodium. An order reads, "500 U/hr IV."

    a. Drop rate/min?

60. Lidocaine hydrochloride 0.4% as continuous IV is ordered for an 80-kg adult to be given at 50 mcg/kg/min.

    a. Amount in mcg/min?

    Using a solution with 4 mg/ml concentration:

    a. Amount to infuse in ml/hr?

    b. Infusion rate in drops/min?

61. Oxytocin 10 U is added to 1 L D5W with orders to infuse at 10 milliunit/min as continuous IV (1000 milliunit = 1 U).

    a. Amount infused in ml/hr?

    b. Drop rate/min?

62. On hand is 1000 ml of D5W containing 4 ml norepinephrine bitartrate resulting in a dilution of 4 mcg/ml. An order is written to give an IV maintenance dose of 4 mcg/min.

    a. Amount in ml/hr?

    b. Drop rate/min?

63. Aminophylline 250 mg in 200 ml D5W is ordered to be given over 8 hours.

    a. Amount in ml/hr?

    b. Amount in mg/hr?

    c. Drop rate/min?

64. Penicillin G potassium 10,000,000 U in 1 L D5W IV is ordered to be given over 12 hours.

    a. Amount of drug in U/ml?

    b. Drop rate/min?

65. A maintenance dose of bretylium tosylate 2 mg/min by continuous infusion IV is ordered. On hand is an ampule of the drug containing 500 mg which is diluted in 500 ml NS.

    a. Amount of drug in mg/ml?

    b. Drop rate/min?

66. Norepinephrine bitartrate 2 mcg/min IV is ordered to follow an initial administration of 8 mcg/min. The IV solution is prepared by adding 4 ml (1 mg/ml) to 1000 ml D5W.

    a. Concentration of drug in mcg/ml?

    b. Amount infused in ml/hr of initial dose?

    c. Amount to be infused in ml/hr of subsequent dose?

67. An IV infusion of regular insulin is prepared by adding 500 U to 500 ml NS. The orders are to give 35 U/hr.

    a. Amount to be given in ml/hr?

    b. Drop rate/min?

68. An IV solution for continuous infusion is prepared by adding 1 Gm lidocaine hydrochloride to 1 L D5W for an order to give 2 mg/min.

    a. Amount of drug in mg/L?

    b. Amount of drug in mg/ml?

    c. Amount to give in drops/min?

69. Potassium chloride (KCl) 15 mEq is added to 500 ml D5W. An order is written to give 2 mEq/hr.

    a. Amount in mEq/ml?

    b. Amount to give in ml/hr?

Using a 10 drop/ml IV solution set, solve problems 70–106.

70. An IV infusion of 2000 ml D5NS is to be given over 16 hours.

    a. Amount infused/hr?

    b. Drop rate/min?

71. An order states that 1250 ml of D2.5W is ordered to be given in 12 hours.

    a. Drop rate/min?

72.   An order states that 300 ml D5W is to be infused in 3 hours.

    a. Drop rate/min?

73.   Five hundred ml of D5W is ordered to be given in 5 hours.

    a. Amount infused/hr?

    b. Drop rate/min?

    c. Number of drops/100 ml?

74.   The physician orders 1 L of D5W to be infused in 8 hours.

    a. Amount infused/hr?

    b. Drop rate/min?

75. Two 1 L bags of D5W followed by 1 L Ringer's Lactate is ordered to be infused over 24 hours.

a. Total amount to be infused in ml?

b. Drop rate/min?

76. One thousand five hundred ml of D5W is adjusted to run at 100 ml/hr.

a. Length of time to infuse total amount?

b. Drop rate/min?

77. A physician orders 1000 ml NS to run at a rate of 20 gtt/min.

a. Amount infused in ml/hr?

b. Length of time to infuse total amount?

78.   An infusion of 1500 ml of D5LR is ordered and started at 4 PM at 20 gtt/min.

a. Completion time for IV?

79.   One L of D5W is ordered to be infused in 10 hours. After 6 hours, 450 ml remain in the bag.

a. Initial drop rate/min?

b. Adjusted drop rate/min?

80.   An order is written to infuse 3 L over 24 hours in the following order: 1 L D5W, 1 L Ringer's Lactate, 1000 ml D5W.

a. Drop rate/min?

After 12 hours, 500 ml of the Ringer's Lactate remain in the second bag.

b. Amount of total left to be infused?

c. Drop rate/min to infuse the remainder?

81. One thousand ml of albumin 5% is hung for an order to administer 500 ml in 2 hours and to administer an additional 500 ml if needed.

    a. Amount in ml/min for first 500 ml?

    b. Drop rate/min?

82. One L of NS is to be infused in 16 hours. Five hundred ml is left after 5 hours.

    a. Amount that should be infused/hr?

    b. Correct drop rate/min?

    c. Actual drop rate/min for first 5 hours?

83. An order for 1000 ml Ringer's Lactate is started at 8 AM to run for 8 hours. The time is 1 PM with 300 ml left in the bottle.

    a. Amount that should have been infused by 1 PM?

    b. Initial drop rate/min?

    c. Adjusted drop rate/min to infuse remaining amount?

84.   One L of D5W is ordered to be given over 24 hours KVO.

a. Drop rate/min?

85.   Five hundred ml of D2.5W is to be infused in 6 hours.

a. Amount infused/hr?

b. Drop rate/min?

86.   An order states that 3000 ml of D5W is to be given in 24 hours.

a. Drop rate/min?

87.   An infusion is running at 20 gtt/min.

a. Amount infused in 8 hours?

88. Two thousand ml of D5W is running at a drop rate/min of 18.

    a. Amount infused/hr?

    b. Length of time to infuse total amount?

89. A patient is to receive D5W at 100 ml/hr.

    a. Amount to give in ml for 4 hours?

    b. Drop rate/min?

90. An order is written to give plasma protein fraction 1.5 L at 2 ml/min.

    a. Length of time to infuse total amount?

    b. Amount infused/hr?

    c. Drop rate/min?

91.   An order of dextran 70 is to be given at 20 ml/kg/24 hr to an adult weighing 154 lb.

   a. Amount to be infused in 24 hours?

   b. Drop rate/min?

92.   Potassium chloride (KCl) 40 mEq in 1 L D5W is started with an order to infuse 2 mEq KCl/hr.

   a. Amount in ml/hr?

93.   An order for plasma protein fraction 250 ml to be given at 5 ml/min.

   a. Amount infused in 15 minutes?

   b. Drop rate/min?

94. Dextran 40, 250 ml has been ordered to be given in 90 minutes.

    a. Amount to be infused in ml/min?

    b. Drop rate/min?

95. Another order of Dextran 40, 250 ml, to be given in 2 hours, followed the above order.

    a. Drop rate/min?

96. Albumin 25%, 100 ml, is to be given IV at 2 ml/min and repeated q2days X 2.

    a. Total amount that will be infused?

    b. Amount infused/30 min?

    c. Drop rate/min?

97.   Dextran 40, 10 ml/kg, is to be infused rapidly for an adult weighing 62 kg.

   a. Amount to be infused?

98.   A continuous IV has been ordered of potassium chloride (KCl) 30 mEq in 1 L D5W. KCl is available in 20 mEq/10 ml and 40 mEq/20 ml.

   a. Which of the available KCl should be used?

   b. Amount of KCl to add to fluid in ml?

   c. Amount infused in mEq if given at 120 ml/hr?

   d. Drop rate/minute if ordered to be given over 10 hours?

99.   KCl for IV injection is available in 60 mEq/30 ml for admixture.

   a. Amount in ml to be added for 40 mEq?

   b. Amount in ml to be added for 30 mEq?

100. Heparin sodium is available in 25,000 U/1000 ml in 0.45% NaCl injection.

    a. Concentration of solution in U/ml?

    The order is to give heparin sodium 2000 U/hr.

    b. Amount to give in ml/hr?

    c. Drop rate/min?

101. Intralipid 10% is ordered to be given at 500 ml over 4 hours. Insert reveals that this should be given at a rate of 1 ml/minute for the first 30 minutes, initially.

    a. Initial drop rate/min?

    b. Drop rate/min after 30 min?

102. Oxytocin 10 U is added to 1000 ml D5RL with orders to infuse 1 milliunit/min as a continuous IV (1000 milliunits = 1 U).

    a. Amount of milliunits/ml?

    b. Amount given in ml/hr?

103.   Morphine sulfate 100 mg is added to 500 ml D5W to be infused at 10 ml/hr.

   a. Amount of drug in mg/ml?

   b. Amount given in mg/hr?

104.   Regular insulin 300 U is ordered IV to be given in 500 ml D5W with orders to give 50 U/hr.

   a. Amount to give in ml/hr?

   b. Drop rate/min?

105.   One L D5NS with 20 mEq KCl is ordered to be given in 12 hours. KCl is available in vials containing 2 mEq/ml.

   a. Amount of KCl to be added in ml?

   b. Drop rate/min?

106. Aminophylline 30 mg/hr is ordered as a continuous IV infusion. Prepared for administration is 500 mg/500 ml in D5W.

    a. Concentration of solution in mg/ml?

    b. Concentration of solution if 500 mg were added to 1 L D5W?

    c. Infusion rate in ml/hr for 500 mg/500 ml?

Refer to Figure 3-3 for problems 107–121.

107. The physician orders packed red cells, 2 units, to be given over 6 hours (250 ml/U).

    a. Amount to be infused/hr?

    b. Drop rate/min?

108. An order states that 500 ml whole blood is to be given over 4 hours (500 ml/U).

    a. Number of units to be given?

    b. Amount in ml/hr?

    c. Drop rate/min?

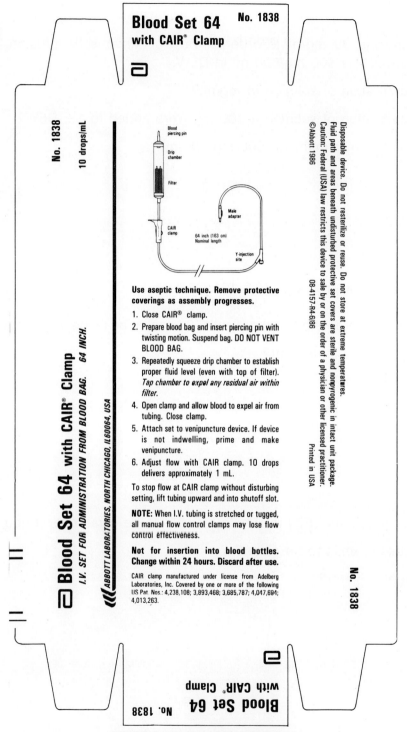

Blood Set 64 No. 1838
with CAIR® Clamp

No. 1838
10 drops/mL

Blood
piercing pin

Drip
chamber

Filter

Male
adapter

CAIR
clamp

64 inch (163 cm)
Nominal length

Y-injection
site

Use aseptic technique. Remove protective coverings as assembly progresses.

1. Close CAIR® clamp.

2. Prepare blood bag and insert piercing pin with twisting motion. Suspend bag. DO NOT VENT BLOOD BAG.

3. Repeatedly squeeze drip chamber to establish proper fluid level (even with top of filter). *Tap chamber to expel any residual air within filter.*

4. Open clamp and allow blood to expel air from tubing. Close clamp.

5. Attach set to venipuncture device. If device is not indwelling, prime and make venipuncture.

6. Adjust flow with CAIR clamp. 10 drops delivers approximately 1 mL.

To stop flow at CAIR clamp without disturbing setting, lift tubing upward and into shutoff slot.

NOTE: When I.V. tubing is stretched or tugged, all manual flow control clamps may lose flow control effectiveness.

Not for insertion into blood bottles. Change within 24 hours. Discard after use.

CAIR clamp manufactured under license from Adelberg Laboratories, Inc. Covered by one or more of the following US Pat. Nos.: 4,238,108; 3,893,468; 3,685,787; 4,047,694; 4,013,263.

Blood Set 64 with CAIR® Clamp
I.V. SET FOR ADMINISTRATION FROM BLOOD BAG. 64 INCH.
ABBOTT LABORATORIES, NORTH CHICAGO, IL 60064, USA

No. 1838

Disposable device. Do not resterilize or reuse. Do not store at extreme temperatures. Fluid path and areas beneath undisturbed protective set covers are sterile and nonpyrogenic in intact unit package. Caution: Federal (USA) law restricts this device to sale by or on the order of a physician or other licensed practitioner.
© Abbott 1986

08-4157-R4-6/86

Printed in USA

Blood Set 64
with CAIR® Clamp

No. 1838

FIGURE 3-3 IV Blood Set; 10 drops/ml
(Reprinted with permission from Abbott Laboratories, Pharmaceutical Products Division)

109.   Two units whole blood is ordered to be given in 12 hours.

   a. Amount given in ml/hr?

   b. Drop rate/min?

110.   Packed red cells, 1 unit, must be given in 4 hours.

   a. Amount in ml/hr?

   b. Drop rate/min?

111.   Four units whole blood are ordered to be given in 12 hours.

   a. Drop rate/min?

112.   Three units of whole blood are to be infused in 12 hours.

   a. Amount in ml/hr?

   b. Drop rate/min?

113.   A unit of whole blood is ordered to be infused at 90 ml/hr.

a. Length of time to infuse total amount?

b. Drop rate/min?

114.   One hundred ml of whole blood is to be infused per hour.

a. Drop rate/min?

115.   Packed red cells, 1 unit, are ordered to be given in 5 hours.

a. Amount to be infused/hour?

b. Drop rate/min?

After 2 hours, 125 ml is left.

c. Adjusted drop rate/min for remaining red cells?

116. The physician orders 2000 ml whole blood to be given in succession over 12 hours. After 3 hours, 1.5 units have been infused.

    a. Amount left to be infused in ml?

    b. Initial drop rate/min?

    c. Adjusted drop rate/min of remaining blood?

117. One unit whole blood is ordered to be given over 6 hours.

    a. Drop rate/min?

118. The physician's order is to give packed red cells, 2 units, in 8 hours.

    a. Amount in ml/hr?

    b. Drop rate/min?

119.   An order states that 125 ml of packed red cells are to be infused per hour.

a. Drop rate/min?

120.   An order of 1500 ml whole blood is to be given over 10 hours.

a. Number of units to be given?

b. Drop rate/min?

121.   Four units of packed red cells are ordered to be given in 24 hours.

a. Drop rate/min?

Refer to Figure 3-4 for problems 122–156.

122. An order is received for an IV infusion of D10W to be given to a neonate at 5 ml/hr.

    a. Amount infused in 24 hr?

    b. Drop rate/min?

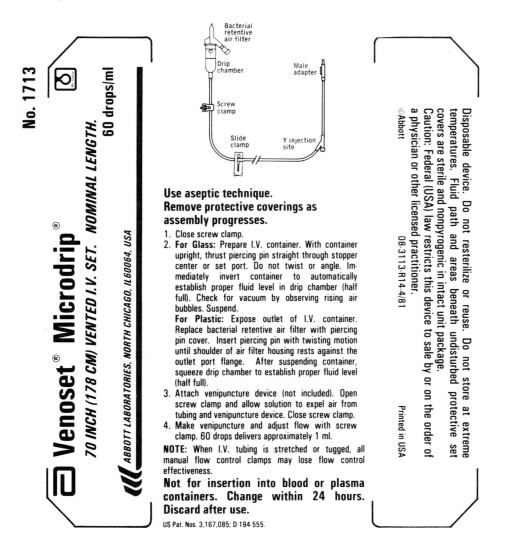

FIGURE 3-4 Venoset Microdrip; 60 drops/ml
(Reprinted with permission from Abbott Laboratories, Pharmaceutical Products Division)

123.   D10W is to be given at 60 ml/kg/24 hr for a neonate weighing 1200 Gm.

a. Weight of neonate in kg?

b. Amount infused in 24 hours?

c. Amount infused/hr?

124.   Five hundred ml of D10W is hung for a term neonate with orders to administer at 14 ml/hr.

a. Amount infused in 24 hours?

b. Drop rate/min?

125.   Orders for an infant state that 100 ml D10W is to be given IV over 4 hours.

a. Amount in ml/hr?

b. Drop rate/min?

126. The order states that an infant is to be infused with 100 ml D10W at 30 gtt/min.

    a. What is the completion time in hours?

127. An infant is to receive 100 ml of D5 in 0.45% NS in 6 hours followed by an additional 200 ml q12h X 2.

    a. Total amount to be infused?

    b. Drop rate/min for first 100 ml?

    c. Drop rate/min for next 24 hours?

128. An IV infusion order for an infant is as follows: 60 ml of 5% protein hydrolysate, 10 ml of dextrose, and 15 ml of NS started at 8 AM and given over 8 hours.

    a. Time for completion of total amount?

    b. Drop rate/min?

129.   A child is to receive 600 ml D5W given in 12 hours.

   a. Drop rate/min?

130.   An order for 250 ml Isolyte M is to be given in 8 hours.

   a. Drop rate/min?

   After 4 hours, 150 ml remain.

   b. Adjusted drop rate/min?

131.   Eighty ml D5W is ordered for a child to be given at 20 drops/min.

   a. Total infusion time?

132.   A child is to be given 750 ml D5W in 24 hours.

   a. Drop rate/min?

133.   A child is to receive D5RL at 30 ml/hour. A 500 ml bag of solution is available to start the IV infusion.

   a. Length of time to infuse 500 ml?

   b. Drop rate/min?

134.   A bag of 250 D5W is hung for a child with orders to infuse at 20 ml/hr.

   a. Drop rate/min?

135.   A 500 ml bag of D5W is to be given over 10 hours.

   a. Amount in ml/hr?

   b. Drop rate/min?

136.   Dextran 40 is ordered to be given at 10 ml/kg/24 hr for a child weighing 88 lb. The dextran comes in 500 ml units.

   a. Weight in kg?

   b. Amount infused in ml/24 hr?

   c. Amount left from available 500 ml unit?

   d. Drop rate/min?

137.   If the order for the above child was for 1 Gm/kg/24 hr and the solution being infused contains 10 Gm/100 ml:

   a. Amount infused in Gm/24 hr?

   b. Amount infused in Gm/hr?

138.   An order for albumin 25% for a 1.4 ml/kg dose is to be given to an infant weighing 1550 Gm.

   a. Weight in kg?

   b. Amount to infused in ml?

139. Plasma protein fraction 22 ml/kg is ordered to be given to a child at 5 ml/min. The child weighs 57 lb.

    a. Weight in kg?

    b. Amount in ml/hr?

    c. Total amount given in ml?

    d. Total infusion time?

    e. If plasma protein fraction comes in 50 mg/ml of protein, what amount of protein is contained in Gm/500 ml?

140. A 250-ml bag of D10W is hung containing potassium chloride (KCl) 5 mEq. The order is for a neonate to receive 120 ml/24 hours.

    a. Amount of KCl in mEq/24 hr?

    b. Amount infused in ml/hr?

141. Potassium chloride is available in 10 mEq/5 ml solution. How much would be needed in ml for an IV of 250 ml D10W containing 5 mEq KCl?

142. A child is to receive 12 mg/kg/24 hr tetracycline hydrochloride divided into 2 doses and given IV in 100 ml D5W over 2 hours. The child's weight is 55 lb.

    a. Total amount in mg/24 hr?

    b. Amount of each dose in mg?

    c. Drop rate/min?

143. A child who weighs 18 kg is to receive 100 mg/kg/24 hr of methicillin sodium IV.

    a. Amount of drug to give in mg/24 hr?

    b. Amount of drug to give in Gm/24 hr?

    The drug is available in 1, 4, and 6 Gm vials.

    c. Which vial is most appropriate to select for dilution?

144.   Amikacin sulfate 165 mg q8h is ordered for a child weighing 34 kg. On hand are vials containing 100 mg/2 ml. Recommended concentration of the drug is 6 mg/ml to be given over 30-60 minutes.

   a. Amount of drug needed in ml?

   b. Total amount needed to produce the recommended dose in ml?

   c. Drop rate/min to infuse in 30 minutes?

145.   A child who weighs 32 kg is to receive phenobarbital sodium 5 mg/kg IV. The maximum dose for 24 hours is 20 mg/kg.

   a. Amount of each dose in mg?

   b. Maximum amount of drug in mg allowed in 24 hours?

   c. Number of doses allowed in 24 hours?

146.   Aminophylline 4 mg/kg as a loading dose followed by 1.3 mg/kg q6h is ordered for a neonate weighing 2 kg. Medication is prepared by the pharmacy in 25 mg/ml dose.

   a. Amount of loading dose in ml?

   b. Amount of each subsequent dose in ml?

147.   Ampicillin sodium 200 mg/24 hr in 2 divided doses is ordered to be given alternately with gentamicin sulfate 4 mg/24 hr in 2 divided doses for a neonate weighing 2000 Gm. Available are ampicillin 200 mg/ml and gentamicin 10 mg/ml preparations.

   a. Weight of neonate in kg?

   b. Amount of ampicillin for each dose in mg?

   c. Amount of ampicillin for each dose in ml?

   d. Amount of gentamicin for each dose in mg?

   e. Amount of gentamicin for each dose in ml?

148.   Mezlocillin sodium 50 mg/kg q4h by IV infusion is ordered for a child weighing 10 kg. The drug is available in 1 Gm vials, each of which is diluted in 10 ml sterile water for injection and then added to 50 ml NS. Orders indicate administration of each dose over 30 minutes by IVPB.

   a. Amount of drug for each dose in mg?

   b. Amount of solution to give for each dose in ml?

   c. Drop rate/min for each dose?

149. Digoxin is available for IV infusion in 0.5 mg/2 ml and 0.1 mg/1 ml. A maintenance dose for a child weighing 20 kg is ordered in the amount of 0.05 mg IV bid.

    a. Which vial should be used to prepare dose?

    b. Amount of each dose in ml?

150. A physician orders cefamandole nafate 250 mg IV injection q8h for a child. The drug is available in 500 mg vials with instructions in the insert to mix each Gm with 10 ml diluent.

    a. Total amount of drug in mg/24 hr?

    b. Amount of diluent to mix with drug in vial?

    c. Amount to give for each dose in ml?

151. An order for a child who weighs 70 lb states that cimetidine 5 mg/kg in 50 ml D5W is to be infused in 60 minutes. The drug is available in 300 mg/2 ml.

    a. Amount of drug to add to the 50 ml?

    b. Drop rate/min?

152.   Penicillin G sodium is available in 5,000,000 U vials. Diluent in the amount of 18 ml is added to a vial to produce a 250,000 U/ml concentration. An order for a child who weighs 80 lb is written to give 50,000 U/kg/24 hr in divided doses to be added to 30 ml D5W q4h IVPB.

   a. Amount in U/24 hr?

   b. Amount in U/dose?

   c. Amount in ml/dose to add to 30 ml solution?

153.   Aminophylline IV of 1 mg/kg/hr is ordered for a child as a maintenance dose. The child weighs 40 lb.

   a. Weight in kg?

   b. Amount in ml/hr for a solution containing 50 mg/500 ml?

154.   The usual dose of furosemide for a child is 2 mg/kg IV.

   a. Amount to give to a child weighing 52 lb?

   b. Amount to give in ml of a solution containing 20 mg/250 ml?

155.   Phenytoin sodium IV is ordered for a child weighing 18 kg. The loading dose ordered is 15 mg/kg.

a. Amount to give in mg?

b. Length of time for infusion if ordered to give at 50 mg/min?

156.   Calculate the drop rates for the following fluids ordered IV for children:

a. 200 ml in 6 hours

b. 500 ml in 8 hours

c. 250 ml in 8 hours

d. 25 ml/hr

e. 40 ml/hr

f. 1200 ml in 24 hours

g. 1000 ml in 24 hours

h. 1000 ml in 18 hours

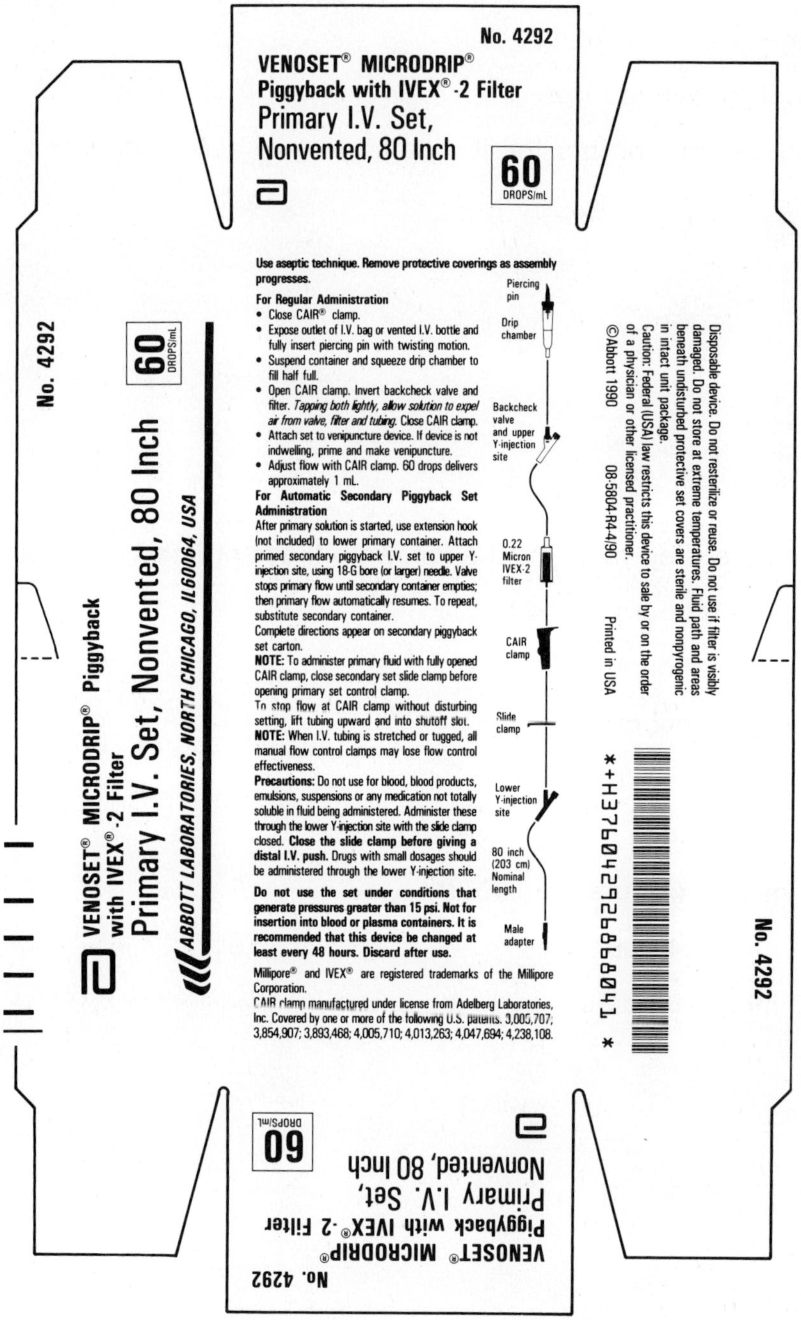
No. 4292
VENOSET® MICRODRIP®
Piggyback with IVEX®-2 Filter
Primary I.V. Set,
Nonvented, 80 Inch
60
DROPS/mL
Use aseptic technique. Remove protective coverings as assembly progresses.
For Regular Administration
• Close CAIR® clamp.
• Expose outlet of I.V. bag or vented I.V. bottle and fully insert piercing pin with twisting motion.
• Suspend container and squeeze drip chamber to fill half full.
• Open CAIR clamp. Invert backcheck valve and filter. Tapping both lightly, allow solution to expel air from valve, filter and tubing. Close CAIR clamp.
• Attach set to venipuncture device. If device is not indwelling, prime and make venipuncture.
• Adjust flow with CAIR clamp. 60 drops delivers approximately 1 mL.
For Automatic Secondary Piggyback Set Administration
After primary solution is started, use extension hook (not included) to lower primary container. Attach primed secondary piggyback I.V. set to upper Y-injection site, using 18-G bore (or larger) needle. Valve stops primary flow until secondary container empties; then primary flow automatically resumes. To repeat, substitute secondary container.
Complete directions appear on secondary piggyback set carton.
NOTE: To administer primary fluid with fully opened CAIR clamp, close secondary set slide clamp before opening primary set control clamp.
To stop flow at CAIR clamp without disturbing setting, lift tubing upward and into shutoff slot.
NOTE: When I.V. tubing is stretched or tugged, all manual flow control clamps may lose flow control effectiveness.
Precautions: Do not use for blood, blood products, emulsions, suspensions or any medication not totally soluble in fluid being administered. Administer these through the lower Y-injection site with the slide clamp closed. Close the slide clamp before giving a distal I.V. push. Drugs with small dosages should be administered through the lower Y-injection site.
Do not use the set under conditions that generate pressures greater than 15 psi. Not for insertion into blood or plasma containers. It is recommended that this device be changed at least every 48 hours. Discard after use.
Millipore® and IVEX® are registered trademarks of the Millipore Corporation.
CAIR clamp manufactured under license from Adelberg Laboratories, Inc. Covered by one or more of the following U.S. patents. 3,005,707; 3,854,907; 3,893,468; 4,005,710; 4,013,263; 4,047,694; 4,238,108.
Piercing pin
Drip chamber
Backcheck valve and upper Y-injection site
0.22 Micron IVEX-2 filter
CAIR clamp
Slide clamp
Lower Y-injection site
80 inch (203 cm) Nominal length
Male adapter
No. 4292
VENOSET® MICRODRIP® Piggyback with IVEX®-2 Filter
Primary I.V. Set, Nonvented, 80 Inch
60 DROPS/mL
ABBOTT LABORATORIES, NORTH CHICAGO, IL60064, USA
Disposable device. Do not resterilize or reuse. Do not use if filter is visibly damaged. Do not store at extreme temperatures. Fluid path and areas beneath undisturbed protective set covers are sterile and nonpyrogenic in intact unit package.
Caution: Federal (USA) law restricts this device to sale by or on the order of a physician or other licensed practitioner.
©Abbott 1990 08-5804-R4-4/90 Printed in USA
No. 4292
VENOSET® MICRODRIP®
Piggyback with IVEX®-2 Filter
Primary I.V. Set,
Nonvented, 80 Inch
60
DROPS/mL
No. 4292

FIGURE 3-5 Venoset Piggyback Microdrip, 60 drops/ml
(Reprinted with permission from Abbott Laboratories Pharmaceutical Products Division)

Refer to Figure 3-5 for problems 157–193.

157. An IV of 250 ml of D5W with 2 mg norepinephrine bitartrate added is prepared for an order to give 8 mcg/min IVPB.

    a. Number of ml containing ordered dose/min?

    b. Drop rate/min?

158. An individual weighing 125 lb is receiving IVPB nitroprusside sodium 50 mg in 500 ml D5W solution with an order to give 2 mcg/kg/min.

    a. Weight in kg?

    b. Amount of drug in mcg in total 500 ml solution?

    c. Amount to give in ml/hr?

    d. Drop rate/min?

159. An order states that 3000 ml NS is to be given over 24 hours. Gentamicin sulfate 80 mg in 100 ml q8h infused over 1 hour IVPB is also ordered.

    a. Drop rate for the primary IV?

    b. Drop rate for the IVPB?

160.   Aminophylline 150 mg in 100 ml D5W is ordered to be given IVPB over 2 hours.

    a. Amount infused in ml/hr?

    b. Drop rate/min?

161.   Isoproterenol hydrochloride is diluted for IV infusion to 1:5000 (0.2 mg/ml) to be given at 2 mcg/min. The solution to be given is prepared by adding 1 mg of the drug to 500 ml D5W.

    a. Amount of drug in mcg/500 ml?

    b. Drop rate/min?

162.   Clindamycin phosphate is available in ampules of 0.6 Gm/4 ml. An order is written to give 300 mg q8h IVPB.

    a. Amount of drug in ml to be added for each administration?

    b. Amount of drug given in mg/24 hr?

163. If the ordered 300 mg dose in problem 162 comes prepared in 50 ml piggyback containers and the dose is to be given over 30 minutes:

    a. Drop rate/min?

164. Cephalothin sodium 500 mg is ordered to be given q6h IVPB. According to the information on the label, Figure 3-6:

    a. Amount of NS to add to the vial?

    b. Amount of drug in mg/24 hr?

    c. Amount of drug in Gm/24 hr?

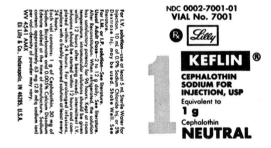

FIGURE 3-6 Keflin (Reprinted with permission from Abbott Laboratories Pharmaceutical Products Division)

165.   Refer to Figure 3-6. If each dose is added to 100 ml D5W to be infused over 1 hour:

   a. Amount of solution from mixture in vial to add to the 100 ml IVPB?

   b. Amount in mg/hr?

   c. Drop rate/min?

166.   Ampicillin sodium 2 Gm in 100 ml IVPB NS is ordered to be given in doses of 1 Gm over 60 min.

   a. Drop rate/min?

167.   The physician orders 1000 ml D5W to be given over 8 hours with ampicillin sodium 0.5 Gm q6h IVPB in 50 ml D5W to be infused over 30 minutes.

   a. Drop rate/min of the 1 L IV?

   b. Drop rate/min of the IVPB?

168. Erythromycin lactobionate 15 mg/kg/24 hr IVPB in divided doses is ordered for a patient who weighs 60 kg. Doses are added to 50 ml D5W to be given q6h over 30 minutes. The drug is available in 500 mg vials with instructions to reconstitute with 10 ml sterile water for injection and then add dose to the 50 ml D5W.

    a. Amount in mg/24 hr?

    b. Amount of reconstituted solution in ml to add for each dose?

    c. Amount in ml/30 min?

    d. Drop rate/min?

169. An order for clindamycin palmitate hydrochloride 300 mg IV in measured container (Volutrol) of D5W to total 50 ml is to be given at a rate of 3 mg/min. The drug is available in 150 mg/ml.

    a. Amount of drug to add in ml?

    b. Amount of D5W in ml?

    c. Amount in ml/hr?

    d. Drop rate/min?

170. An order for aminophylline 200 mg in 50 ml D5W IVPB is to be given over 1 hour. On hand is 500 mg/20 ml vial.

    a. Amount of drug in mg/ml in vial?

    b. Amount of drug needed in ml?

    c. Total amount of IV solution?

    d. Drop rate/min?

171. A stat order states that 400 mg aminophylline in 50 ml D5W IVPB is to be given over 60 minutes. 500 mg/25 ml is available.

    a. Amount of available drug to use in ml?

    b. Total amount of solution in ml?

    c. Drop rate/min?

172. Vials of aminophylline 500 mg/20 ml and nafcillin sodium solution 1 Gm/50 ml D5W are on hand. The orders are to give 750 mg aminophylline in 1 L D5W at 20 mg/hr and 500 mg nafcillin q4h IVPB via heparin lock.

    a. Amount of aminophylline to be added to 1 L in ml?

    b. Amount to infuse to give 20 mg/hr in ml?

    c. Amount of nafcillin to give for each dose in ml?

    d. Total amount of nafcillin/24 hr in mg?

173. Methicillin sodium 1 Gm q6h IVPB is ordered. Each dose is diluted in 100 ml NS and given at a rate of 10 ml/min. According to the information on the label, Figure 3–7:

    a. Amount of diluent to add to give 10 mg/ml?

    b. Amount of each dose in mg?

    c. Amount of drug in mg/ml?

    e. Total amount of drug given in mg/24 hr?

    e. Drop rate/min?

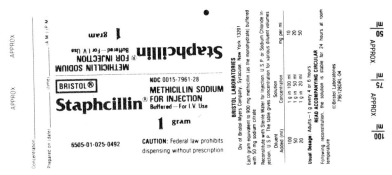

FIGURE 3–7 Staphcillin (Reprinted with permission from Eli Lilly and Company)

174. Cefamandole nafate 1 Gm in 200 ml D5W q12h IVPB is ordered to be administered over 3 hours.

    a. Total amount of each dose in ml?

    b. Drop rate/min?

175.   An IV infusion of 1000 ml D5W stopped dripping with 200 ml remaining in the primary line and 20 ml remaining in the IVPB medication line.

    a. How long would it take to give the remaining solutions if the drop rate/min is set at 20 gtt/min?

176.   Procainamide hydrochloride 2 mg/min is ordered IVPB. On hand is a solution of 0.5 Gm/250 ml D5W.

    a. Amount of drug in mg/ml?

    b. Drop rate/min?

177.   An order for 2 L D5W given over 24 hours is written. In addition, cefazolin sodium 1 Gm in 100 ml D5W IVPB q8h is to be given over 1 hour. According to the information on the label, Figure 3-8:

    a. Amount of drug in vial?

    b. Amount of diluent to add to reconstitute the drug?

    c. Total volume in vial after reconstitution in ml and mg?

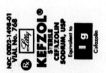

CAUTION—Federal (U.S.A.) law prohibits dispensing without prescription.
    For I.M. or I.V. Use
    Dosage—See Literature
To prepare solution add 2.5 mL Sterile
Water for Injection.
SHAKE WELL   Protect from Light
Provides an approximate volume of
3.0 mL (330 mg per mL)
Prior to Reconstitution: Store at Con-
trolled Room Temperature 59° to 86°F
(15° to 30°C)
After reconstitution: Store in a refriger-
ator. For Storage Time - See Accom-
panying Literature. If kept at room tem-
perature, use within 24 hours.
       Lyophilized
WV 4531 AMX
  Eli Lilly & Co., Indianapolis, IN 46285, U.S.A.

FIGURE 3-8 Kefzol 1 g (Reprinted with permission from Bristol-Myers Pharmaceutical Group)

178. For the administration of cefazolin sodium in problem 177:

    a. Amount to be added to IVPB for each dose?

    b. Amount of drug infused in mg/ml?

    c. Total amount in ml/24 hr?

179. Tetracycline hydrochloride is available in 150 mg and 500 mg vials for IV use. The order is for 250 mg q12h diluted in 150 ml D5W to be given over 2 hours. Five ml diluent is added to reconstitute the drug before adding it to the IVPB container of 150 ml.

    a. Amount infused in mg/ml?

    b. Amount infused in ml/hr?

    c. Drop rate/min?

180. Amphotericin B 1 mg/250 ml D5W IVPB is ordered.

    a. Drop rate/min if ordered to be given over 6 hours?

181.   An order for piperacillin sodium 2 Gm q4h IVPB is written. The drug is on hand in 4 Gm vials and piggyback solution sets of 50 or 100 ml. The insert directs that the drug should be diluted in 1 Gm/5 ml for IV use and then added to 50 ml and given over 30 minutes.

a. Amount of diluent to be added in ml?

b. Amount in ml to be added to the piggyback?

c. Total amount in IVPB to be given in ml?

d. Drop rate/min?

182.   A physician orders nafcillin sodium 500 mg q4h for 24 hours by heparin lock to be given over 30 minutes as intermittent IV. On hand are 500 mg vials and piggyback fluid in 50 and 100 ml volumes. The insert advises to add 1.7 ml diluent to each 500 mg vial resulting in 2 ml nafcillin solution.

a. Total amount in ml of each IVPB infusion?

b. Total amount of drug in mg/24 hr?

c. Drop rate/min if dose is added to 50 ml piggyback?

183. Chloramphenicol sodium succinate 1 Gm/10 ml when mixed is available for administration of an IV order to give 50 mg/kg/24 hr in 4 equal doses to an individual weighing 80 kg.

    a. Amount of each dose in mg?

    After diluting the drug according to directions in 50 ml diluent:

    b. Amount in ml to give for each dose?

    c. Drop rate/min if given over 60 min?

184. Nitroprusside sodium is available for injection in 50 mg vials. A solution is prepared by mixing the contents of the vial with 3 ml D5W. The order is written to add this to 500 ml D5W and administer 3 mcg/kg/min via IV secondary line with 1 L KVO primary line. The individual's weight is 60 kg.

    a. Amount of drug in mg/ml?

    b. Amount of drug in mcg/ml?

    c. Amount to give in mcg/min?

    d. Amount to give in ml/hr?

185. Methylprednisolone sodium succinate 200 mg is ordered to be given q6h IVPB. Each dose is diluted in 50 ml solution according to the insert directions.

    a. Drop rate/min if given over 30 minutes?

    b. Drop rate/min if given over 90 minutes?

186. Doxapram hydrochloride 1 mg/minute by IV infusion via secondary line is ordered. The solution for the IV is prepared by adding 400 mg to 180 ml solution. The medication is available in 20 mg/ml vials.

  a. Amount in ml of drug to add to 180 ml solution?

  b. Concentration of solution in mg/ml?

  c. Amount to give in ml/min?

187. Moxalactam disodium 4 Gm/24 hours in divided doses q12h IVPB is ordered. On hand are 2 Gm vials. Directions state to dilute each 2 Gm in 10 ml diluent and then add to 100 ml D5LR with each dose to be given over 2 hours.

  a. Number of vials needed for each dose?

  b. Amount in ml of each dose?

  c. Drop rate/min?

188. Nitroglycerin is available in 25 mg vials with concentration of 5 mg/ml. The contents of a vial is added to 500 ml diluent to carry out an order to administer 5 mcg/minute IV.

  a. Concentration in mcg/ml of total IV?

  b. Amount to give in ml/hr?

  c. Drop rate/min?

189. If the contents in problem 188 are added to 300 ml diluent:

    a. Concentration in mcg/ml?

    b. Amount to give in ml/hr?

    c. Drop rate/min?

190. An individual weighing 190 lb has an order for dopamine hydrochloride 5 mcg/kg/min IVPB. The solution available contains 200 mg/250 ml D5W.

    a. Weight in kg?

    b. Concentration of solution in mg/ml?

    c. Concentration in mcg/ml?

    d. Amount to give in mcg/min?

    e. Drop rate/min?

191. An order is written for quinidine gluconate 200 mg IVPB to be administered at 1 ml/minute. The medication is prepared by using 80 mg/ml in a 10 ml vial added to 40 ml D5W.

    a. Total volume of prepared solution in ml?

    b. Amount of drug in the 10 ml vial in mg?

    c. Amount of drug administered in mg/min?

    d. Amount of time to administer prescribed dose in minutes?

192. Cefoxitin sodium 1 Gm q6h IVPB is ordered. The medication after reconstitution results in 2 Gm/21 ml vials. Each dose is prepared by adding the ordered amount of medication to a 50 ml solution.

a. Amount in ml to add for each dose?

b. Drop rate/min to give each dose in 30 minutes?

193. Ritodrine hydrochloride 150 mg is added to 500 ml NS to equal 0.3 mg/ml for an order to give 0.1 mg/minute, not to exceed 120 mg/24 hr.

a. Amount to give in ml/min?

b. Drop rate/min?

Perform the calculations for the following single-dose IV problems (194-234).

194. A single dose of factor IX complex 75 units/kg is ordered to be given IV to an individual weighing 110 lb.

a. Weight in kg?

b. Amount to give in units?

195. Prednisolone sodium phosphate 15 mg q12h IV injection is ordered. The drug is available in 20 mg/ml vials.

    a. Number of vials needed for doses/24 hr?

    b. Amount of each dose in ml?

196. Glucagon 0.5 mg IV is ordered with the dose to be repeated in 5–20 minutes if no response. Drug is available in 1 mg and 10 mg vials and is reconstituted with a diluent supplied with the vial.

    a. Which vial should be used?

    b. Which vial should be used if 1 mg/dose is ordered?

197. Heparin sodium 5000 U bolus is ordered as an initial dose by direct IV to be followed by a continuous IV infusion. On hand is a vial containing 10,000 U/ml.

    a. Amount to give in ml?

    b. Amount to give in U?

198.   A single dose of metoclopramide hydrochloride 10 mg IV is ordered. The medication is available in 10 mg/2 ml vials.

   a. Amount to give in ml?

   An order of 2.5 mg IV of this drug is to be given to a child.

   b. Amount to give in ml?

199.   Furosemide 1 mg/kg IV is ordered for an individual weighing 155 lb with an increase in dosage by 1 mg/kg in 2 hours following the initial dose.

   a. Amount of each dose in mg?

200.   Metaraminol bitartrate is available in 10 mg/ml vials. Five ml of the drug has been added to 500 ml LR for IV administration.

   a. Amount of drug added in mg?

   b. Concentration of solution in mg/500 ml?

   c. Concentration of solution in mg/ml?

   If the initial dose of 5 mg is ordered by direct injection:

   d. Amount to give in ml?

201. Isoproterenol hydrochloride is available for injection in a 1:5000 concentration which is equal to 0.2 mg/ml. The solution for an IV injection is prepared by diluting 1 ml of the concentration in 9 ml D5W. The order is to give 0.02 mg.

    a. Amount of diluted solution to give in ml?

202. An order is written for lidocaine hydrochloride bolus IV of 50 mg given at the rate of 20 mg/minute, with repeat if indicated but with a limit of 200 mg/hr allowed.

    a. Amount of time to give initial dose?

    b. Amount of time to give initial and one repeat dose?

203. Morphine sulfate 10 mg IV is to be given over 5 minutes. The preparation for injection contains 10 mg/5 ml.

    a. Amount to give in ml?

    b. Amount in mg/ml?

204.   An order for antihemophilic factor 250 U to be given by IV injection qAM is written as a prophylactic measure for an individual weighing 50 kg. The usual dose is 10–30 U/kg.

    a. Amount given in U/kg?

    b. Is this amount less or more than the usual dosage?

    c. Range of correct amount in U for this individual?

205.   Cimetidine 300 mg q8h IV is ordered. The drug is available in 300 mg/2 ml vials. The amount allowed in 24 hours is 2400 mg.

    a. Amount of each dose in ml?

    b. Total amount in mg/24 hr?

    c. Additional amount in mg allowed in 24 hr?

206.   A digitalizing dose of digoxin 10 mcg/kg by direct IV injection is ordered for an individual weighing 132 lb.

    a. Weight in kg?

    b. Amount given in mcg?

    c. Amount given in mg?

207. Ethacrynate sodium 0.5 mg/kg is ordered to be given by direct injection and administered slowly to an individual weighing 54 kg. A maximum single dose should not exceed 100 mg.

    a. Amount to give in mg?

    b. Amount to give in mg if order is for 1 mg/kg?

    c. Does either dose exceed the maximum?

208. Nalbuphine hydrochloride 10 mg q3h IV prn is ordered. Ampules of 10 mg/ml are available.

    a. Possible total amount in mg/24 hr?

    b. Amount of each dose in ml?

209. An order states, ''Naloxone hydrochloride 1.5 mg IV stat and may repeat q2–3 minutes up to 10 mg.'' Ampules containing 1 mg/ml are available.

    a. Amount of each dose in ml?

    b. Number of times drug may be repeated?

210.   An order is written for a single dose of undiluted glycopyrrolate 0.1 mg. According to the information on the label, Figure 3-9:

   a. Total amount in vial in ml?

   b. Amount of drug in mg/ml?

   c. Amount to be given in ml?

211.   Metoclopramide hydrochloride 10 mg IV as a single dose to be given over 2 minutes is ordered. According to the information on the label, Figure 3-10:

   a. Amount of drug in each ml?

   b. Amount of drug to give in ml?

   c. Total amount of drug in vial in mg/ml?

212.   A repeat dose of verapamil hydrochloride 10 mg IV is to be given over 2 minutes. According to the information on the label, Figure 3-11:

   a. Amount of drug to give in ml?

   b. Amount of drug to give in ml/30 sec?

NDC 0031-7890-83 *A·H·ROBINS*
20 ml MULTIPLE DOSE VIAL
Robinul® Injectable
(Glycopyrrolate Injection, USP)
0.2 mg/ml
Water for Injection, USP q.s./Benzyl
Alcohol, NF (preservative) 0.9%.
pH adjusted, when necessary, with hydro-
chloric acid and/or sodium hydroxide.
NOT FOR USE IN NEWBORNS

CAUTION: Federal law prohibits dispens-
ing without prescription.
For intramuscular or intravenous adminis-
tration.
For dosage and other directions for use,
consult accompanying product literature.
Store at Controlled Room Temperature,
Between 15°C and 30°C (59°F and 86°F).
MANUFACTURED FOR PHARMACEUTICAL DIVISION
A. H. ROBINS COMPANY, RICHMOND, VA. 23220
by ELKINS-SINN, INC., CHERRY HILL, N.J. 08003
a subsidiary of A. H. Robins   10.87

FIGURE 3-9 Robinul 0.2 mg/ml (Reprinted with permission from A. H. Robins Co.)

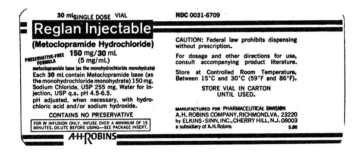

FIGURE 3-10 Reglan 150 mg/30 ml (Reprinted with permission from A. H. Robins Co.)

NDC 0044-1815-11 4mL
ISOPTIN®
verapamil HCl
INTRAVENOUS
10 mg/4 mL
Knoll Pharmaceuticals
Whippany, NJ 07981

FIGURE 3-11 Isoptin 10 mg/4 ml (Reprinted with permission from Knoll Pharmaceuticals)

213.   Colchicine 2 mg IV as an initial dose with 0.5 mg q6h to follow is to be administered over 5 minutes by direct injection. According to the information on the label, Figure 3-12:

a. Amount contained in mg/ml?

b. Amount in ml needed for the initial dose?

c. Amount in ml needed for subsequent doses?

d. Total amount of drug in mg/24 hr including initial dose?

e. Total amount of drug in ml/24 hr to be given?

f. Amount of drug given in mg/min of initial dose?

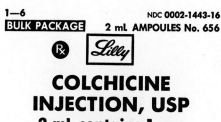

FIGURE 3-12 Colchicine 1 mg/2 ml (Reprinted with permission from Eli Lilly and Company)

214. The colchicine in problem 213 is diluted in NS for IV administration by combining 1 ampule with 5 ml NS.

    a. Amount of initial dose in ml?

    b. Amount of subsequent doses in ml?

215. An IV bolus of regular insulin 0.33 U/kg is ordered for an adult weighing 138 lb. According to the information on the label, Figure 3-13:

    a. Amount of insulin in U/ml?

    b. Amount of insulin to give in U?

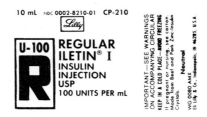

FIGURE 3-13 Iletin I Insulin 100 U/ml (Reprinted with permission from Eli Lilly and Company)

216. Metoprolol tartrate 5 mg IV bolus q2min for up to 3 doses is ordered. According to the information on the label, Figure 3-14:

    a. Amount of drug for each dose in ml?

    b. Total amount of drug allowed in mg?

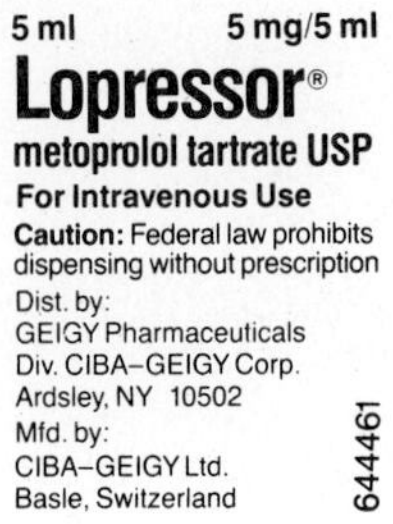

5 ml   5 mg/5 ml

Lopressor®

metoprolol tartrate USP

For Intravenous Use

Caution: Federal law prohibits
dispensing without prescription

Dist. by:
GEIGY Pharmaceuticals
Div. CIBA–GEIGY Corp.
Ardsley, NY 10502
Mfd. by:
CIBA–GEIGY Ltd.
Basle, Switzerland

644461

FIGURE 3–14 Lopressor 5 mg/5 ml (Reprinted with permission from CIBA-GEIGY Corp.)

217. Sodium bicarbonate 1 mEq/kg IV bolus is ordered with additional 0.5 mEq/kg q10min for an individual weighing 85 kg. The solution provided for the IV contains 50 mEq/50 ml.

    a. Amount in mEq for initial bolus administration?

    b. Amount in ml for initial bolus?

    c. Amount in mEq for each additional dose?

    d. Amount in ml for each additional dose?

218. Atropine sulfate 0.01 mg/kg IV is ordered for an individual weighing 121 lb, to be given over 1 minute. According to the information on the label, Figure 3-15:

    a. Amount of drug to give in mg?

    b. Amount to give in ml?

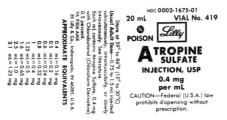

FIGURE 3-15 Atropine Sulfate (Reprinted with permission from Eli Lilly and Company)

219. An order is written for aminophylline 225 mg IV bolus per heparin lock. The drug on hand is labeled 25 mg/ml. The order states that bolus should be given at the rate of 25 mg/min.

    a. Amount of drug to give in ml?

    b. Amount of time to give dose in minutes?

220. An IV bolus of meperidine hydrochloride 30 mg is ordered and 50 mg/ml is available.

    a. Amount to give in ml?

    b. Amount of time if order reads to limit rate to 10 mg/min?

221.   Digoxin 0.350 mg is ordered IV push to be given at a rate of 0.5 mg/min using a solution containing 0.25 mg/ml.

   a. Amount of drug to give in ml?

   b. Amount of time to give ordered dose?

222.   The physician orders diazepam 5 mg/minute as IV bolus as an initial dose with repeat dose q15min of up to 30 mg. The drug is available in 10 mg/ml vials.

   a. Amount of each dose in ml?

   b. Number of doses allowed including the initial dose?

223.   Vincristine sulfate 0.01 mg/kg IV to be given over 1 minute is ordered for an individual weighing 88 lb.

   a. Weight in kg?

   b. Amount to give in mg?

224. An IV injection of nafcillin sodium 750 mg q4h is ordered. The drug is available in 500 mg and 1 Gm vials. Instructions are to dilute in 30 ml sterile water for injection and give over 10 minutes.

    a. Which vial should be selected?

    b. Amount of solution in ml to give for each dose?

225. Methoxamine hydrochloride 5 mg is ordered to be injected slowly IV. The drug is available in 20 mg/ml vials.

    a. Amount to give in ml?

226. Iron dextran is available for injection in 50 mg/ml vials. An order for 100 mg IV daily is written.

    a. Amount to give in ml?

227. Heparin sodium 50 U/kg as an initial dose is ordered for a child weighing 62 lb.

    a. Amount to give in U?

228.   Benzquinamide hydrochloride 25 mg IV is ordered to be given at the rate of 1 ml over 1 minute. Each ml contains 25 mg of the drug.

a. Amount of time to give the dose?

229.   An intermittent IV injection of heparin sodium 5000 U q6h is ordered. Available are two vials: 20,000 U/1 ml and 20,000 U/2 ml.

a. Which vial would be selected?

b. Amount in ml to give for each dose using the 2 ml vial?

c. Total amount in U/24 hr?

d. Total amount in ml/24 hr?

230.   Bretylium tosylate undiluted 5 mg/kg by rapid injection IV is ordered for an individual weighing 60 kg. Vials containing 50 mg/ml are available.

a. Amount of the dose in mg?

b. Amount to give in ml?

231. Diazoxide 1 mg/kg as IV bolus with orders to repeat q5–15min as needed up to a maximum of 150 mg is to be given. On hand are vials of 300 mg/20 ml. The adult patient weighs 121 lb.

    a. Weight in kg?

    b. Amount in mg for each dose?

    c. Amount in ml of each dose using the vial on hand?

232. Azathioprine sodium is ordered in an initial dose of 5 mg/kg daily for an individual weighing 80 kg.

    a. Amount in mg of each dose?

    Maintenance doses of 3 mg/kg daily IV is ordered following the initial regimen.

    b. Amount in mg of each dose?

    The drug is available in 100 mg vials.

    c. Number of vials needed for initial dose?

    d. Number of vials needed for daily maintenance dose?

233.   Labetalol hydrochloride 20 mg as direct IV injection is ordered to be given over 2 minutes. The solution concentration to be used is 10 mg/10 ml.

   a. Amount to give in ml?

234.   Famotidine 20 mg q12h is ordered to be given by IV injection over 2 minutes. Available for use is 10 mg/ml per vial. The directions in the insert advise using each vial with 5 ml diluent.

   a. Amount in each vial after dilution?

   b. Total amount in ml for each dose?

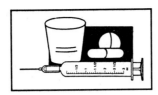

ANSWER KEY

MATHEMATICS REVIEW

Review Set 1

1. $\frac{6}{6}$, $\frac{7}{5}$

2. $\frac{1}{100}$
   $\frac{1}{150}$

3. $\frac{1}{4}$, $\frac{1}{14}$

4. $1\frac{2}{9}$, $1\frac{1}{4}$, $5\frac{7}{8}$

5. $\frac{3}{4} = \frac{6}{8}$, $\frac{1}{5} = \frac{2}{10}$
   $\frac{3}{9} = \frac{1}{3}$

6. $\frac{13}{2}$

7. $\frac{6}{5}$

8. $\frac{32}{3}$

9. $\frac{47}{6}$

10. $\frac{411}{4}$

11. 2

12. 1

13. $3\frac{1}{3}$

14. $1\frac{1}{3}$

15. $2\frac{3}{4}$

16. $\frac{6}{8}$

17. $\frac{4}{16}$

18. $\frac{8}{12}$

19. $\frac{4}{10}$

20. $\frac{6}{9}$

21. $\frac{1}{100}$

22. $\frac{1}{10,000}$

23. $\frac{5}{9}$

24. $\frac{3}{10}$

Solutions – Review Set 1

8. $10\frac{2}{3} = (3 \times 10) + 2 = \frac{32}{3}$

14. $\frac{100}{75} = 1\frac{25}{75} = 1\frac{1}{3}$

18. $\frac{2}{3} \times \frac{4}{4} = \frac{8}{12}$

Review Set 2

1. $\frac{1}{40}$

2. $\frac{36}{125}$

3. $\frac{35}{48}$

4. $\frac{3}{100}$

5. 3

6. $8\frac{7}{15}$

7. $1\frac{5}{12}$

8. $17\frac{5}{24}$

9. $1\frac{1}{24}$

10. $32\frac{5}{6}$

11. $\frac{1}{2}$

12. $4\frac{5}{6}$

13. $\frac{1}{24}$

14. $66\frac{23}{33}$

15. $299\frac{4}{5}$

16. $\frac{1}{30}$

17. $3\frac{1}{3}$

18. $\frac{3}{20}$

19. $\frac{1}{3}$

20. $1\frac{1}{3}$

Solutions – Review Set 2

3. $\dfrac{5}{8} \times 1\dfrac{1}{6} = \dfrac{5}{8} \times \dfrac{7}{6} = \dfrac{35}{48}$

5. $\dfrac{\frac{1}{6}}{\frac{1}{4}} \times \dfrac{3}{\frac{2}{3}} = \dfrac{1}{6} \times \dfrac{4}{1} = \dfrac{2}{3}$

$3 \times \dfrac{3}{2} = \dfrac{9}{2}$

$\dfrac{\cancel{2}}{\cancel{3}} \times \dfrac{\cancel{9}}{\cancel{2}} = 3$

8. $4\dfrac{2}{3} + 5\dfrac{1}{24} + 7\dfrac{1}{2} = 4\dfrac{16}{24}$

$5\dfrac{1}{24}$

$+ 7\dfrac{12}{24}$

$16\dfrac{29}{24} = 17\dfrac{5}{24}$

14.
$$100\dfrac{1}{33} \qquad 99\dfrac{34}{33}$$
$$- 33\dfrac{1}{3} \qquad - 33\dfrac{11}{33}$$
$$\overline{\qquad\qquad} \qquad \overline{66\dfrac{23}{33}}$$

17. $2\dfrac{1}{2} \div \dfrac{3}{4} = \dfrac{5}{2} \div \dfrac{3}{4} = \dfrac{5}{\cancel{2}} \times \dfrac{\cancel{4}}{3} =$

$\dfrac{10}{3} = 3\dfrac{1}{3}$

20. $\dfrac{\frac{3}{4}}{\frac{7}{8}} \div \dfrac{1\frac{1}{2}}{2\frac{1}{3}} = \left(\dfrac{3}{\cancel{4}} \times \dfrac{\cancel{8}}{7}\right) \div \left(\dfrac{3}{2} \times \dfrac{3}{7}\right) =$

$\dfrac{6}{7} \div \dfrac{9}{14} = \dfrac{\cancel{6}}{\cancel{7}} \times \dfrac{\cancel{14}}{\cancel{9}} = \dfrac{4}{3} = 1\dfrac{1}{3}$

Review Set 3

1. 0.2, two-tenths

2. $\dfrac{17}{20}$, 0.85

3. $1\dfrac{1}{20}$, one and five-hundredths

4. $\dfrac{3}{500}$, six-thousandths

5. 10.015, ten and fifteen-thousandths

6. $1\dfrac{9}{10}$, one and nine-tenths

7. $5\dfrac{1}{10}$, 5.1

8. 0.8, eight-tenths

9. $250\dfrac{1}{2}$, two hundred fifty and five-tenths

10. 33.03, thirty-three and three hundredths

11. $\dfrac{19}{20}$, ninety-five hundredths

12. 2.75, two and seventy-five hundredths

13. $7\dfrac{1}{200}$, 7.005

14. 0.084, eighty-four thousandths

15. $12\dfrac{1}{8}$, twelve and one hundred twenty-five thousandths

16. $20\dfrac{9}{100}$, twenty and nine-hundredths

Review Set 3 (cont.)

17. $22\frac{11}{500}$, 22.022

18. $\frac{3}{20}$, fifteen-hundredths

19. 1000.005, one thousand and five-thousandths

20. $4085\frac{3}{40}$, 4085.075

Solutions – Review Set 3

4. $\frac{6}{1000} = \frac{3}{500}$

8. $\frac{4}{5} = 5)\overline{4.0}^{\,0.8}$

14. $\frac{21}{250} = 250)\overline{21.000}^{\,0.084}$
   $\underline{20\ 00}$
   $1\ 000$
   $\underline{1\ 000}$

15. $12.125 = 12\frac{125}{1000} = 12\frac{1}{8}$

18. $0.15 = \frac{15}{100} = \frac{3}{20}$

Review Set 4

1. 22.585
2. 44.177
3. 12.309
4. 11.3

5. 175.199
6. 25.007
7. 0.518
8. $9.48

9. $18.91
10. $22.71
11. 6.403
12. 0.27

13. 4.15
14. 1.51
15. 10.25
16. 2.517

17. 374.35
18. 604.42
19. 27.449
20. 23.619

Solutions – Review Set 4

2. 7.517
    3.200
    0.160
    $\underline{33.300}$
    44.177

9. $\overset{8\ 9\ 10}{\$19.00}$
    $\underline{-\ 0.09}$
    $18.91

Review Set 5

1. 5.83
2. 2.2
3. 42.75
4. 0.15
5. 403.14
6. 75,100.75

7. $32.86
8. $2.78
9. 348.58
10. 0.02
11. 400
12. 3.74

13. 5
14. 2.98
15. 4120
16. $5.45
17. $272.67
18. 1.5

19. 50,020
20. $300
21. 562.50. = 56,250
22. 16.0. = 160
23. .025. = 0.025
24. .032.005 = 0.032005

Review Set 5 (cont.)

25. .00.125 = 0.00125
26. 23.2.5 = 232.5
27. 71.7.717 = 71.7717
28. 83.1.6 = 831.6
29. 0.33. = 33
30. 14.106. = 14,106

Solutions – Review Set 5

10. 1.14 × 0.014 = 0.01596 = 0.02   14. 45.5 ÷ 15.25 = 2.983 = 2.98

Review Set 6

1. 0.4, 40%, 2:5   6. 0.17, 17%, 1:6   11. 0.67, $\frac{2}{3}$, 67%   16. 0.3, $\frac{3}{10}$, 30%

2. $\frac{1}{20}$, 5%, 1:20   7. 0.5, $\frac{1}{2}$, 1:2

12. 0.33, 33%, 1:3   17. 0.02, 2%, 1:50

3. 0.17, $\frac{17}{100}$, 17:100   8. 0.01, $\frac{1}{100}$, 1%   13. $\frac{13}{25}$, 52%, 13:25   18. $\frac{3}{5}$, 60%, 3:5

4. 0.25, $\frac{1}{4}$, 25%   9. $\frac{9}{100}$, 9%, 9:100   14. 0.45, $\frac{9}{20}$, 45%   19. $\frac{1}{25}$, 4%, 1:25

5. 0.06, $\frac{3}{50}$, 3:50   10. 0.38, 38%, 3:8   15. 0.86, 86%, 6:7   20. 0.1, $\frac{1}{10}$, 1:10

CHAPTER 1

1. 1/2 tab   7. 5 ml   13. 2 tab
2. 1 tab   8. 1/2 tab   14. 2 tab
3. 1/2 tab   9. 1 tab   15. a) 764 mg
4. 1 tab   10. 1 1/2 tab   b) 3056 mg
5. 2 tab   11. 18.75 mg   16. 1 tab
6. 2 tab   12. 1/2 tab   17. 45 ml

18. 1 cap

19. 1/2 tab

20. 1 cap

21. 2 tab

22. a) 7.5 ml
    b) 1 1/2 tsp

23. 2 cap

24. 1 1/2 tab

25. 1 tab

26. a) 1 oz
    b) 2 tbsp
    c) 30 ml

27. 2 tab

28. 1 cap

29. 1 cap

30. a) 0.2 Gm per dose
    b) 1.2 Gm per day

31. 2 tab

32. 1 tab

33. 1 cap

34. 1 tab

35. 2 tab

36. a) 2 mg
    b) 10 ml
    c) 2 tsp

37. 1/2 tab

38. 2 tab

39. 1 cap

40. 1 cap

41. 1 tab

42. 1 tsp

43. 2 tab

44. a) 2 1/2 tsp
    b) 12.5 ml

45. 1 tab

46. 1/2 tab

47. gr 1/4

48. 2 tab

49. a) 500,000 U
    b) 5 ml

50. 20 Gm

51. 1 tab

52. a) 1/3 oz
    b) 10 ml

53. 2 tab

54. 2 tab

55. 2 tsp

56. a) 80 mg
    b) 4 ml

57. 2 tab

58. 2 tab

59. 1 tab

60. 1/2 tab

61. 1 tab

62. 2 cap

63. 15 ml

64. 2 cap

65. a) gr 3/4
    b) gr iii

66. 2.5 ml

67. 1 tab

68. 5 ml

69. 2 tab

70. 2 cap

71. 2 tab

72. 1 ml

73. 2 tab

74. a) 10 ml
    b) 2 tsp

75. 1/2 of 300 mg tab

76. a) 1020 mg minimum
    b) 1700 mg maximum

77. 1 tab

78. 10 ml

79. 2 tab

80. 1 tab

81. 2 tab

82. 2 tab

83. 1/2 tab

84. 5 ml

85. 1 tab

86. 1 tab

87.   4 ml

88.   1 tab

89.   288 mg

90.   5 ml

91.   2 tab

92.   16 Gm

93.   1/2 tab

94.   1 1/2 cap

95.   2 tab

96.   2 tab

97.   2 tab

98.   15 ml

99.   16 ml

100. 1 tab

101. 10 ml

102. 3 tab

103. 1 cap

104. 1.5 Gm

105. 5 ml

106. 1 cap

107. 2 cap

108. 0.1 Gm

109. a) 1 tab
      b) 3 tab

110. 1/2 tab

111. a) 100 mg
      b) 20 ml
      c) 4 tsp

112. 2 cap

113. a) 2 cap
      b) 1200 mg

114. 4 tsp

115. 2 cap

116. 2 cap

117. a) 2 cap
      b) 1 cap

118. 1 each 5 mg tab +
      1 each 10 mg tab
      OR 1 1/2 10 mg tab

119. a) 2 tab
      b) gr $\dot{+}$

120. 5 ml

121. 2 cap

122. 12 ml

123. a) 30 mg minimum
      b) 48 mg maximum

124. a) 15 ml
      b) 1 tbsp
      c) 1/2 oz

125. 3000 mg

126. 1.5 Gm

127. 2 tab

128. a) 2 tab
      b) 8 tab

129. 2 tab

130. 1 tab

131. 1 cap

132. 2 cap

133. 4 cap

134. 1 cap

135. 1/2 tab

136. 2 tab

137. 5 ml

138. a) 2 tsp
      b) 10 ml

139. 15 ml

140. 2 tab

141. 1 1/2 tab

142. 2 tab

143. 2 tab

144. 2 tab

145. a) 200 mg
      b) 5 ml

146. 2 tab

147. a) 3 tab
      b) 1 tab

148. a) yes
      b) 1 tab

149. 1 1/2 tab

150. 2 tab

151. 2 tab

152. a) 100 mg
      b) 1 tab

153. 5 ml

154. 3 cap
155. 1 cap
156. a) 1000 mg
  b) 10 ml
157. gr 1/15
158. 2 tab
159. 3 tab
160. 1/2 of 250 mg tab
161. 20 ml
162. 1 cap
163. 2 tab
164. 1 0.05 mg tab
165. 1 tab
166. 1 1/2 tab
167. 2 tab
168. 2 tab
169. a) 1/2 tab
  b) gr ＋

170. 1/2 oz
171. 2 tab
172. 1.25 ml
173. 1 tab
174. 1/2 tab
175. 1 tab
176. 2 tab
177. a) 30 ml
  b) 10 ml
178. 2 tab
179. 1 1/2 tab
180. 2 tab
181. 1/2 tab
182. a) 2 tab
  b) 10 ml
183. 1/2 tab
184. 2 tab
185. 2 tab

186. 2 tab
187. a) 0.4 Gm
  b) 2 cap
188. 1 1/2 tab
189. 1/2 tab
190. 2 tab
191. a) 550 mg
  b) 275 mg
192. a) 2 cap
  b) gr s̄s̄
193. 2 tab
194. 1 cap
195. 1 tab
196. 2 pulvules
197. 2 tab
198. 5 ml
199. 1000 mg
200. gr VIIs̄s̄

CHAPTER 2

1. 100%
2. 350 mg
3. 2 ml
4. 1 ml
5. 0.5 ml
6. 2 ml

7. a) 45 mg minimum
  b) 72 mg maximum
8. 2 ml
9. 2 ml
10. 1.25 ml
11. 3 ml
12. 1 ml

13. 0.75 ml
14. 0.7 ml
15. 2 ml
16. 1.5 ml
17. 2 ml
18. 0.5 ml

19. 2 ml

20. 2 ml

21. 0.3 ml

22. 0.5 ml

23. 2 ml

24. 2 amp

25. 0.5 ml

26. a) 16.5 U
     b) 33 U

27. 3 m

28. 2 ml

29. 8 m

30. 2 ml

31. 0.5 ml

32. 2 ml

33. 1.5 ml

34. 2 ml

35. 0.5 ml

36.

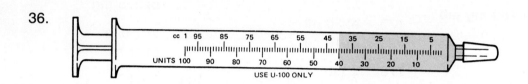

37. 0.4 ml

38. 2 ml

39. 1 ml

40. 1.5 ml

41. 1.25 ml

42. 2.5 ml

43. 5 ml

44. 30 U isophane insulin and 15 U regular insulin

45. 2 ml

46. 1.6 mg

47. 0.5 ml

48. 1.5 ml

49. 1.5 ml

50. 1 ml

51. a) yes
     b) 2 ml

52. 0.25 ml

53. a) 14 doses
     b) 3 m

54. 0.75 ml

55. 3.3 ml

56. 1 ml

57. 1.9 ml

58. 0.5 ml

59. 2.25 ml

60. 2 ml

61.

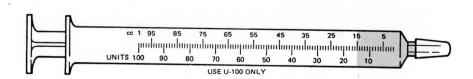

62. 2 ml	67. a) 33 mg b) 0.7 ml	72. 5 ml
63. 1.5 ml	68. 1 Gm	73. 0.5 ml
64. 1 ml	69. 3 ml	74. 2 ml
65. 2 ml	70. 0.8 ml	75. 0.2 mg
66. 2 ml	71. 6 m	76. 0.6 ml

77.

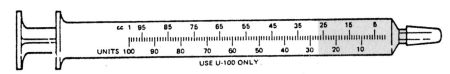

78. 0.2 ml

79. 2.5 mg

80. 0.7 ml

81. 1.2 ml

82. 0.75 ml

83. 1.2 ml

84.

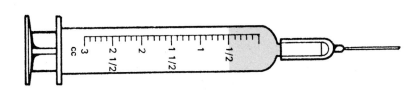

85.

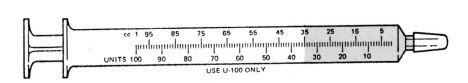

86.	2 ml	92.	2 ml	98.	3 ml
87.	2 ml	93.	gr 1/300	99.	1.1 ml
88.	8 mg	94.	2 ml	100.	0.4 ml
89.	0.8 ml	95.	1 ml	101.	1.9 ml
90.	28 U	96.	2 ml	102.	1 ml
91.	1.4 ml	97.	4 m	103.	3 ml

104.

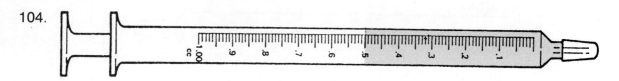

105.	0.2 ml	120.	2 ml	134.	8 m
106.	1.5 ml	121.	2 ml	135.	0.5 ml
107.	0.75 ml	122.	0.5 ml	136.	2 ml
108.	0.5 ml	123.	0.75 ml	137.	0.6 ml
109.	1.5 ml	124.	a) 52.5 mg	138.	0.5 ml
110.	0.5 ml		b) 0.7 ml	139.	0.75 ml
111.	0.8 ml	125.	2 ml	140.	0.5 ml
112.	2.25 ml	126.	0.5 ml	141.	1.8 ml
113.	0.25 ml	127.	1.5 ml	142.	0.2 ml
114.	0.5 ml	128.	0.2 ml	143.	1.3 ml
115.	3 ml	129.	1 ml	144.	0.25 ml
116.	1.5 ml	130.	2 ml	145.	0.28 Gm
117.	2 ml	131.	1 ml	146.	0.75 ml
118.	0.4 ml	132.	2 ml	147.	0.4 ml
119.	0.5 Gm	133.	0.7 ml	148.	0.7 ml

149. 1.5 ml

150. 2 ml

151. 0.4 ml

152. 25 U

153. 0.6 ml

154. 2 ml

155. 0.75 ml

156. 0.8 ml

157. a) 2.25 ml
     b) 3 ml

158. 0.5 ml

159. 0.9 ml

160. 1.5 ml

161.

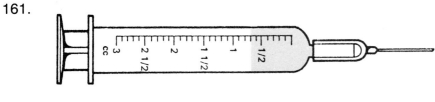

162.

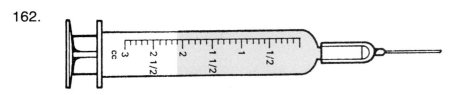

163.

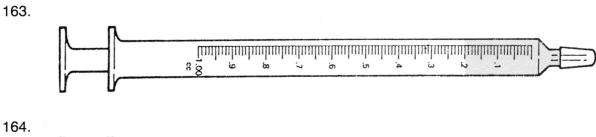

164.

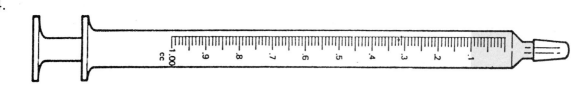

165.

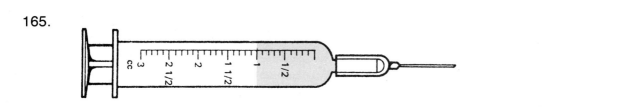

166.

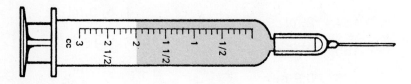

167. a) 420 mcg

b)

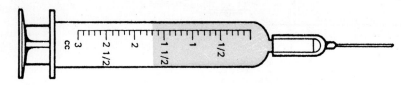

168.

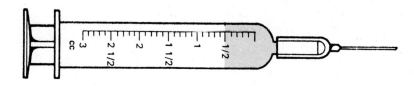

169.

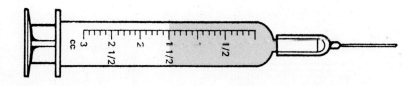

170. a) 0.05 Gm

b)

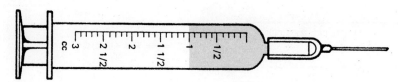

CHAPTER 3

1. a) 100 ml/hr
   b) 25 gtt/min

2. a) 125 ml/hr
   b) 31 gtt/min

3. a) 10 gtt/min

4. a) 83 ml/hr
   b) 21 gtt/min

5. a) 21 gtt/min

6. a) 2 L
   b) 28 gtt/min

7. a) 3 L or 3000 ml
   b) 25 hr
   c) 30 gtt/min

8. a) 100 ml/hr
   b) 800 ml/8 hr

9. a) 25 gtt/min
   b) 31 gtt/min

10. a) 5 hours as order
    is written
    b) 25 gtt/min

11. a) 420 ml/5 hr

12. a) 31 gtt/min
    b) 21 gtt/min

13. a) 94 ml/hr
    b) 23 gtt/min

14. a) 25 gtt/min

15. a) 21 gtt/min

16. a) 25 gtt/min
    b) 400 ml

c) 700 ml
d) 50 gtt/min (more
   than accepted
   25% increase in
   rate)

17. a) 8 AM
    b) 31 gtt/min

18. a) 31 gtt/min

19. a) 1000 ml/8 hours
    b) 31 gtt/min

20. a) 31 gtt/min

21. a) 2.5 L
    b) 26 gtt/min

22. a) 1400 ml by 8 PM
    b) 1333 ml by 8 PM
    c) 28 gtt/min
    d) 25 gtt/min

23. a) 50 gtt/min
    b) No, should have
       infused at 21
       gtt/min or 21 ml/15
       min

24. a) 12 mEq
    b) 31 gtt/min

25. a) 63 ml/hr
    b) 1500 ml
    c) 16 gtt/min

26. a) 360 ml/hr
    b) 90 gtt/min

27. a) 1250 U/hr
    b) 10 gtt/min

28. a) 50 U/ml
    b) 20 ml/hr

29. a) 1 mg/ml
    b) 20 ml/hr

30. a) 120 ml/hr
    b) 30 gtt/min

31. a) 10 ml/hr
    b) 3 gtt/min

32. a) 500 ml/12 hr
    b) 1667 U/hr
    c) 10 gtt/min

33. a) 580 ml

34. a) 4000 mcg/ml
    b) 7.7 ml/min

35. a) 25 mcg/ml
    b) 12 ml/hr

36. a) 83 ml/hr
    b) 83 gtt/min

37. a) 83 gtt/min

38. a) 42 ml/hr
    b) 42 gtt/min

39. a) 42 gtt/min

40. a) 63 gtt/min

41. a) 12 hours
    b) 75 gtt/min

42. a) 50 ml/hr
    b) 20 hours

43. a) 25 ml/hr
    b) 25 gtt/min

44. a) 360 ml/6 hr
    b) 60 gtt/min

45. a) 31 gtt/min

46. a) 100 gtt/min

47. a) 125 gtt/min

48. a) 2500 ml or 2.5 L
    b) 104 gtt/min

49. a) 151 ml/6 hr

50. a) 6 PM
    b) 100 gtt/min

51. a) 0.4 mg/ml
    b) 7.5 ml/hr
    c) 7.5 gtt/min

52. a) 65 kg
    b) 325 ml/hr

53. a) 50 ml

54. a) 49.5 mcg/ml
    b) 12 ml/hr
    c) 12 gtt/min

55. a) 60 kg
    b) 1 mg/ml
    c) 30 ml/hr
    d) 30 gtt/min

56. a) 1 mg/ml
    b) 45 ml/hr

57. a) 25 U/ml
    b) 40 gtt/min

58. a) 50 U/ml
    b) 10 ml/hr
    c) Increase 1 ml/hr for
       each 50 U added

59. a) 50 gtt/min

60. a) 4000 mcg/min
    b) 60 ml/hr
    c) 60 gtt/min

61. a) 60 ml/hr
    b) 60 gtt/min

62. a) 60 ml/hr
    b) 60 gtt/min

63. a) 25 ml/hr
    b) 31.3 mg/hr
    c) 25 gtt/min

64. a) 10,000 U/ml
    b) 83 gtt/min

65. a) 1 mg/ml
    b) 120 gtt/min

66. a) 4 mcg/ml
    b) 120 ml/hr
    c) 30 ml/hr

67. a) 35 ml/hr
    b) 35 gtt/min

68. a) 1000 mg/L
    b) 1 mg/ml
    c) 120 gtt/min

69. a) 0.03 mEq/ml
    b) 67 ml/hr

70. a) 125 ml/hr
    b) 21 gtt/min

71. a) 17 gtt/min

72. a) 17 gtt/min

73. a) 100 ml/hr
    b) 17 gtt/min
    c) 1000 gtt/100 ml

74. a) 125 ml/hr
    b) 21 gtt/min

75. a) 3000 ml
    b) 21 gtt/min

76. a) 15 hours
    b) 17 gtt/min

77. a) 120 ml/hr
    b) 8 hours and 20
       minutes

78. a) 4:30 AM

79. a) 17 gtt/min
    b) 19 gtt/min

80. a) 21 gtt/min
    b) 1500 ml
    c) 21 gtt/min

81. a) 4 ml/min
    b) 42 gtt/min

82. a) 63 ml/hr
    b) 10 gtt/min
    c) 17 gtt/min

83. a) 625 ml by 1 PM
    b) 21 gtt/min
    c) 17 gtt/min

84. a) 7 gtt/min

85. a) 83 ml/hr
    b) 14 gtt/min

86. a) 21 gtt/min

87. a) 960 ml/8 hr

88. a) 108 ml/hr
    b) 18 hours and 31
       minutes

89. a) 400 ml/4 hr
    b) 17 gtt/min

90. a) 12 hours and 30 minutes
    b) 120 ml/hr
    c) 20 gtt/min

91. a) 1400 ml/24 hr
    b) 10 gtt/min

92. a) 50 ml/hr

93. a) 75 ml/15 min
    b) 50 gtt/min

94. a) 2.8 ml/min
    b) 28 gtt/min

95. a) 21 gtt/min

96. a) 300 ml
    b) 60 ml/30 min
    c) 20 gtt/min

97. a) 620 ml

98. a) Use 40 mEq/20 ml since need is for 30 mEq
    b) 15 ml
    c) 3.6 mEq
    d) 17 gtt/min

99. a) 20 ml
    b) 15 ml

100. a) 25 U/ml
     b) 80 ml/hr
     c) 13 gtt/min

101. a) 10 gtt/min
     b) 22 gtt/min

102. a) 10 milliunits/ml
     b) 6 ml/hr

103. a) 0.2 mg/ml
     b) 2 mg/hr

104. a) 30 ml/hr
     b) 5 gtt/min

105. a) 10 ml
     b) 14 gtt/min

106. a) 1 mg/ml
     b) 0.5 mg/ml
     c) 30 ml/hr

107. a) 83 ml/hr
     b) 14 gtt/min

108. a) 1 unit
     b) 125 ml/hr
     c) 21 gtt/min

109. a) 83 ml/hr
     b) 14 gtt/min

110. a) 63 ml/hr
     b) 10 gtt/min

111. a) 28 gtt/min

112. a) 125 ml/hr
     b) 21 gtt/min

113. a) 5 hours and 34 minutes
     b) 15 gtt/min

114. a) 17 gtt/min

115. a) 50 ml/hr
     b) 8 gtt/min
     c) 7 gtt/min

116. a) 1250 ml left
     b) 28 gtt/min
     c) 23 gtt/min

117. a) 14 gtt/min

118. a) 63 ml/hr
     b) 10 gtt/min

119. a) 21 gtt/min

120. a) 3 units
     b) 25 gtt/min

121. a) 7 gtt/min

122. a) 120 ml/24 hr
     b) 5 gtt/min

123. a) 1.2 kg
     b) 72 ml/24 hr
     c) 3 ml/hr

124. a) 336 ml/24 hr
     b) 14 gtt/min

125. a) 25 ml/hr
     b) 25 gtt/min

126. a) 3 hours and 20 minutes

127. a) 500 ml
     b) 17 gtt/min
     c) 17 gtt/min

128. a) 4 PM
     b) 11 gtt/min

129. a) 50 gtt/min

130. a) 31 gtt/min
     b) 38 gtt/min

131. a) 4 hours

132.   a) 31 gtt/min

133.   a) 16 hours and 40
        minutes
        b) 30 gtt/min

134.   a) 20 gtt/min

135.   a) 50 ml/hr
        b) 50 gtt/min

136.   a) 40 kg
        b) 400 ml/24 hr
        c) 100 ml left
        d) 17 gtt/min

137.   a) 40 Gm/24 hr
        b) 1.67 Gm/hr

138.   a) 1.55 kg
        b) 2.2 ml

139.   a) 26 kg
        b) 300 ml/hr
        c) 572 ml total
        d) 1 hour and 54
           minutes
        e) 25 Gm/500 ml

140.   a) 2.4 mEq/24 hours
        b) 5 ml/hr

141.   a) 2.5 ml

142.   a) 300 mg/24 hr
        b) 150 mg/dose
        c) 50 gtt/min

143.   a) 1800 mg/24 hr
        b) 1.8 Gm/24 hr
        c) 2 of the 1 Gm vials
           would be needed

144.   a) 3.3 ml
        b) 27.5 ml
        c) 55 gtt/min

145.   a) 160 mg
        b) 640 mg/24 hr
        c) 4 doses

146.   a) 0.32 ml
        b) 0.1 ml

147.   a) 2 kg
        b) 100 mg/dose
        c) 0.5 ml/dose
        d) 2 mg/dose
        e) 0.2 ml/dose

148.   a) 500 mg/dose
        b) 30 ml/dose
        c) 60 gtt/min

149.   a) 0.1 mg/1 ml
        b) 0.5 ml/dose

150.   a) 750 mg/24 hr
        b) 5 ml
        c) 2.5 ml/dose

151.   a) 1.06 ml
        b) 50 gtt/min

152.   a) 1,800,000 U/24
           hr
        b) 300,000 U/dose
        c) 1.2 ml/dose

153.   a) 18 kg
        b) 1.8 ml/hr

154.   a) 48 mg/dose
        b) 3.8 ml

155.   a) 270 mg
        b) 5 hours and 24
           minutes

156.   a) 33 gtt/min
        b) 63 gtt/min
        c) 31 gtt/min
        d) 25 gtt/min
        e) 40 gtt/min
        f) 50 gtt/min
        g) 42 gtt/min
        h) 56 gtt/min

157.   a) 1 ml/min
        b) 60 gtt/min

158.   a) 57 kg
        b) 50,000 mcg/500 ml
        c) 68 ml/hr
        d) 68 gtt/min

159.   a) 125 gtt/min
        b) 100 gtt/min

160.   a) 50 ml/hr
        b) 50 gtt/min

161.   a) 1000 mcg/500 ml
        b) 60 gtt/min

162.   a) 2 ml
        b) 900 mg/24 hr

163.   a) 100 gtt/min

164.   a) 10 ml stated on
           label
        b) 2000 mg/24 hr
        c) 2 Gm/24 hr

165.   a) 5 ml
        b) 500 mg/hr
        c) 105 gtt/min

166.   a) 50 gtt/min

167.   a) 125 gtt/min
        b) 100 gtt/min

168. a) 900 mg/24 hr
b) 4.5 ml
c) 54.5 ml/30 min
d) 109 gtt/min

169. a) 2 ml
b) 48 ml
c) 30 ml/hr
d) 30 gtt/min

170. a) 25 mg/ml
b) 8 ml
c) 58 ml
d) 58 gtt/min

171. a) 20 ml
b) 70 ml
c) 70 gtt/min

172. a) 30 ml
b) 27 ml/hr
c) 25 ml/dose
d) 3000 mg/24 hr

173. a) 100 ml on label for 10 mg/ml
b) 1000 mg/dose
c) 10 mg/ml
d) 4000 mg/24 hr
e) 120 gtt/min

174. a) 200 ml
b) 67 gtt/min

175. a) 11 hours for both

176. a) 2 mg/ml
b) 60 gtt/min

177. a) 1 Gm on label
b) 2.5 ml diluent
c) 3.0 ml and 330 mg/ml

178. a) 3 ml added to each dose to give 1 Gm
b) 10 mg/ml
c) 2300 ml/24 hr

179. a) 1.6 mg/ml
b) 78 ml/hr
c) 78 gtt/min

180. a) 41 gtt/min

181. a) 20 ml
b) 10 ml to IVPB
c) 60 ml
d) 120 gtt/min

182. a) 52 ml or 102 ml
b) 3000 mg/24 hr
c) 104 gtt/min

183. a) 1000 mg/dose
b) 60 ml/dose
c) 60 gtt/min

184. a) 10.1 mg/ml
b) 10,100 mcg/ml
c) 180 mcg/min
d) 1.2 ml/hr

185. a) 100 gtt/min
b) 33 gtt/min

186. a) 20 ml
b) 2.2 mg/ml
c) 0.5 ml/min

187. a) A 2 Gm vial/dose
b) 110 ml
c) 55 gtt/min

188. a) 49.5 mcg/ml
b) 6 ml/hr
c) 6 gtt/min

189. a) 82 mcg/ml
b) 3.7 ml/hr
c) 4 gtt/min

190. a) 86 kg
b) 0.8 mg/ml
c) 800 mcg/ml
d) 430 mcg/min
e) 32 gtt/min

191. a) 50 ml
b) 800 mg
c) 16 mg/min
d) 12.5 min

192. a) 10.5 ml
b) 121 gtt/min

193. a) 0.33 ml/min
b) 20 gtt/min

194. a) 50 kg
b) 3750 units

195. a) 2 vials/24 hr
b) 0.75 ml/dose

196. a) 1 mg vial
b) 1 mg vial for each dose

197. a) 0.5 ml
b) 5000 U as ordered

198. a) 2 ml
b) 0.5 ml

199. a) 70.5 mg

200. a) 50 mg
b) 50 mg/500 ml
c) 0.1 mg/ml
d) 0.5 ml

201.   a) 1 ml

202.   a) 2.5 minutes
        b) 5 minutes

203.   a) 5 ml
        b) 2 mg/ml

204.   a) 5 U/kg
        b) Less than usual
           dose
        c) 500-1500 U

205.   a) 2 ml
        b) 900 mg/24 hr
        c) 1500 mg

206.   a) 60 kg
        b) 600 mcg
        c) 0.6 mg

207.   a) 27 mg
        b) 54 mg
        c) Neither exceed
           100 mg

208.   a) 80 mg/24 hr
        b) 1 ml/dose

209.   a) 1.5 ml
        b) 5-6 repeat doses

210.   a) 20 ml vial
        b) 0.2 mg/ml
        c) 0.5 ml

211.   a) 5 mg/ml
        b) 2 ml
        c) 150 mg/30 ml

212.   a) 4 ml to give 10 mg
        b) 1 ml/30 sec

213.   a) 1 mg/2 ml
        b) 4 ml
        c) 1 ml
        d) 4 mg/24 hr
        e) 8 ml/24 hr
        f) 0.4 mg/min

214.   a) 14 ml/dose
        b) 3.5 ml/dose

215.   a) 100 U/ml
        b) 20.7 U

216.   a) 5 mg/5 ml on label
           so 5 ml/dose
        b) 15 mg

217.   a) 85 mEq
        b) 85 ml
        c) 42.5 mEq
        d) 42.5 ml

218.   a) 0.55 mg
        b) 1.4 ml

219.   a) 9 ml
        b) 9 minutes

220.   a) 0.6 ml
        b) 3 minutes

221.   a) 1.4 ml
        b) .7 min

222.   a) 0.5 ml
        b) 6 doses

223.   a) 40 kg
        b) 0.4 mg

224.   a) 1 Gm vial for 750
           mg/dose
        b) 22.5 ml/dose

225.   a) 0.25 ml

226.   a) 2 ml

227.   a) 1400 U

228.   a) 1 minute since 25
           mg ordered to be
           given over 1 minute
           from 25 mg/ml

229.   a) Either vial will
           supply 20,000 U/24
           hr
        b) 0.5 ml
        c) 20,000 U/24 hr
        d) 2 ml/24 hr

230.   a) 300 mg/dose
        b) 6 ml/dose

231.   a) 55 kg
        b) 55 mg/dose
        c) 3.7 ml/dose

232.   a) 400 mg/dose
        b) 240 mg/dose
        c) 4 vials of 100 mg
           each
        d) 3 vials for 240 mg

233.   a) 20 ml

234.   a) 6 ml
        b) 12 ml/dose